PERINATOLOGY

Nestlé Nutrition Workshop Series
Volume 26

PERINATOLOGY

Editor

Erich Saling, M.D.
Professor of Obstetrics and Perinatal Medicine
Institut für Perinatale Medizin
der Freien Universität Berlin
Berlin, Germany

NESTLÉ NUTRITION SERVICES

RAVEN PRESS ■ NEW YORK

Nestec Ltd., 55 Avenue Nestlé, CH-1800 Vevey, Switzerland
Raven Press, Ltd., 1185 Avenue of the Americas, New York,
New York 10036

Made in the United States of America

Library of Congress Cataloging-in-Publication Data

Perinatology / editor, Erich Saling.
     p.   cm. — (Nestlé Nutrition workshop series ; v. 26)
    Based on the 26th Nestlé Nutrition Workshop held in Berlin, Germany, May 14–16, 1990.
    Includes bibliographical references and index.
    ISBN 0-88167-822-8
    1. Perinatology—Congresses. I. Saling, Erich. II. Nestlé Nutrition Workshop (26th : Berlin, Germany : 1990) III. Series.
    [DNLM: 1. Fetal Monitoring—congresses. 2. Perinatology— congresses. 3. Pregnancy Complications. Infections—congresses. 4. Prenatal Diagnosis—congresses. W1 NE228 v. 26 / WQ 210 P4483 1990]
RG600.P43   1991
618.3'2—dc20
DNLM/DLC
for Library of Congress   91-18567

9 8 7 6 5 4 3 2 1

Preface

Three factors give the 26th Nestlé Workshop held in Berlin special significance, one of which has particular personal importance.

First, Berlin is regarded by various perinatologists as the cradle of modern perinatal medicine, or, to put it more correctly, of *pre*natal medicine. It was here in 1960 that the initial steps were taken in fetal blood analysis (1), enabling the first direct diagnostic approach to the human fetus, which, apart from primitive auscultation of the fetal heart, was not possible up to that time. Other important events in Berlin were the founding of the first national society of perinatal medicine in 1967, and a year later the first international association of perinatal medicine, the European Association. These facts provide a historical logic as to why a Nestlé Workshop specifically about perinatology should take place in Berlin.

The second factor was not in existence when the meeting was originally planned but has emerged as a result of the recent political upheavals. Following the political breakdown in eastern Europe, Berlin has become a center of action, and since the Wall was opened, it has been a world-wide symbol of peaceful revolution for freedom.

The third factor is a personal one. This is the last important international scientific meeting that I conducted during my official professional career, for I shall retire from my academic post this year. However, I intend to remain scientifically active in the institute that I have built up, though with the status of an emeritus.

The large field of prenatal medicine—an important part of perinatal medicine—has only emerged during the last 30 years. I enjoy comparing its exceptional progress in obstetric history with the concurrent advances in space exploration. In a way previously unthinkable, we have gained medical access to our own small cosmic space, the human "breeding space."

Within the framework of this workshop we shall be dealing with a few selected topics taken from this huge new field that touches many other medical disciplines. Sadly, even rapid progress soon becomes a matter of routine. Thus, it is important for us to remember that we, the generation alive today, are direct witnesses to a remarkable epoch that contained so many achievements in perinatal medicine.

ERICH SALING, M.D.
Berlin, Germany

REFERENCE

1. Saling E. Fetal blood analysis. In: Rooth G, Saugstad OD, eds. *The roots of perinatal medicine.* Stuttgart: Thieme, 1985.

Acknowledgments

I would like to express my thanks to all those who have participated in this workshop. My special thanks are extended to the Nestlé Company, in particular to Dr. Pierre Guesry and Dr. Laïla Dufour from Vevey, Switzerland, and to Mr. Betz, Mr. Hoffmann, and Mr. Lutz from Frankfurt and Munich, for having chosen Berlin as the venue for the 26th Workshop.

Foreword

Perinatalogy was chosen as the subject for the 26th Nestlé Nutrition Workshop for "historical" reasons, because 22 years ago the Nestlé Company sponsored the first European Congress of Perinatal Medicine, at the time when this new medical branch—linking obstetrics and pediatrics—first appeared. In 1968 the president of that Congress was Professor Erich Saling, one of the pioneers of fetal examination during the prenatal period, and he is the chairman of this workshop.

Since then far greater progress has been made than could ever have been imagined at the onset, and progress continues today. A few key subjects were selected, because of either their great importance or their innovative aspect.

We have not limited ourselves strictly to the "perinatal" period as originally defined, partly because some fetal exploratory techniques must be carried out at an early stage of gestation, and partly because embryonic and early fetal diagnostic techniques are among the most important recent developments.

Our aim is to present advances in this field, contributed by experts from all over the world, knowing that a greater understanding of technical progress by multi-disciplinary teams is indispensable (to enable them to give better care to the child and better advice and help to the family). A more complete title of the seminar and this volume would be "Prenatal and Perinatal Medicine: Progress and Future Outlook; Selected Topics."

We hope that this book contributes to the diffusion of knowledge to all those involved in fetal and neonatal care and also in child care in general, obstetricians, pediatricians, and other specialists, not only because of the data it contains on technical progress but also for the information it gives on the evolution of practical aspects of perinatalogy and on research paths for the future.

Laïla Dufour-Khouri, M.D.
*Assistant to the Medical
and Scientific Director
Nestec Ltd., Vevey, Switzerland*

Contents

Role of Infections in Late Abortions and Prematurity

Contributors

Geoffrey S. Dawes
Nuffield Department of Obstetrics
  and Gynaecology
University of Oxford
John Radcliffe Hospital
Oxford OX3 9DU, United Kingdom

David A. Eschenbach
Department of Obstetrics and
  Gynecology, RH-20
University of Washington
Seattle, Washington 98195, USA

Tetsuro Fujiwara
Department of Pediatrics
Iwate Medical University School of
  Medicine
Uchimaru 19-I
Morioka 020, Iwate, Japan

Mitchell S. Golbus
Department of Obstetrics, Gynecology
  and Reproductive Sciences
University of California, San Francisco
School of Medicine
San Francisco, California 94143-0720,
  USA

Karl-Heinz Grzeschik
Abteilung für Allgemeine Humangenetik
Medizinisches Zentrum für
  Humangenetik der Universität
  Marburg
Bahnhofstrasse 7a
D-3550 Marburg, Germany

Calvin J. Hobel
Division of Maternal-Fetal Medicine
Cedars-Sinai Medical Center
8700 Beverly Boulevard
Los Angeles, California 90048-0750,
  USA

Wolfgang Holzgreve
Department of Obstetrics and
  Gynecology
Zentrum für Frauenheilkunde
Westfälische Wilhelms-Universität
Albert-Schweitzer Strasse 33
D-4400 Münster, Germany

Peter Hope
Department of Paediatrics
John Radcliffe Hospital
Oxford OX3 9DU, United Kingdom

Ian R. Johnson
Department of Obstetrics and
  Gynaecology
City Hospital
Hucknall Road
Nottingham NG5 1PB, England

Pentti Jouppila
Department of Obstetrics and
  Gynecology
University of Oulu
90220 Oulu, Finland

Asim Kurjak
Ultrasonic Institute
University of Zagreb
"Dr. Josip Kajfes" Hospital
Pavleka Miskine 64
41000 Zagreb, Yugoslavia

Dietrich W. Roloff
Department of Pediatrics
L-3023/0254
University of Michigan Hospitals
Ann Arbor, Michigan 48109, USA

Karl G. Rosén
Division of Perinatal Physiology
Department of Physiology
University of Göteborg
Box 330 31
400 33 Göteborg, Sweden

Erich Saling
Institut für Perinatale Medizin der
Freien Universität Berlin
Abteilung für Geburtsmedizin der
Frauenklinik Berlin-Neukölln
Mariendorfer Weg 28
D-1000 Berlin 44, Germany

Stephan Schmidt
Department of Gynecology and
Obstetrics
University of Bonn
Universitäts-Frauenklinik
Venusberg
Sigmund Freud Strasse 25
5300 Bonn 1, Germany

Herman P. Van Geijn
Department of Obstetrics and
Gynecology
Free University Hospital
P.O. Box 7057
1007 MB Amsterdam, The Netherlands

Invited Attendees

Dachrul Aldy / *Medan, Indonesia*
Asril Aminullah / *Jakarta,*
Indonesia
Djauhariah Arifuddin Madjid /
Ujung Pandang, Indonesia
O. A. Bremer / *Stuttgart,*
Germany
M. Caccamo / *Milan, Italy*
M. Carstensen / *Hamburg,*
Germany
Fong-Ming Chang / *Tainan,*
Taiwan, R.O.C.
M. Elser / *Landshut, Germany*
M. Faber / *Leipzig, Germany*
A. Feige / *Nürnberg, Germany*
M. Frenzel / *Jena, Germany*
M. Fricke / *Würzburg, Germany*
Francis Gold / *Tours, France*
M. Grauel / *Berlin, Germany*
M. Gröbe / *Nürnberg, Germany*
M. Heller / *Ludwigsburg,*
Germany
Sunthorn Horpaopan / *Bangkok,*
Thailand
M. Hoyme / *Essen, Germany*
Mostéfa Keddari / *Alger, Algeria*
Robert Küchler / *Berlin, Germany*

Volker Lehmann / *Hamburg,*
Germany
Pierre Lequien / *Lille, France*
Antonio Marini / *Milan, Italy*
M. Martius / *Würzburg, Germany*
Alex Mathews / *Johor Bahru,*
Malaysia
M. Menzel / *Erfurt, Germany*
R. H. Merchant / *Bandra*
Bombay, India
Michael Obladen / *Berlin,*
Germany
Chairuddin Panusunan Lubis /
Medan, Indonesia
Birgit Peitersen / *Hvidovre,*
Denmark
Arnold Pollak / *Vienna, Austria*
M. Robel / *Leipzig, Germany*
Hellfried Rosegger / *Graz, Austria*
Erwin Sarwono / *Surabaya,*
Indonesia
R. Schäfer / *Hamm, Germany*
Rainer Schilling / *St. Pölten,*
Austria
M. Schwarzenau / *Berlin,*
Germany

Walter Stögmann / *Vienna, Austria*

Ramen Subramaniam / *Kuala Lumpur, Malaysia*

Ranjit Laxman TambyRaja / *Singapore, Singapore*

Yulniar M. Tasli / *Palembang, Indonesia*

Iskandar Wahidiyat / *Jakarta, Indonesia*

M. Wauer / *Berlin, Germany*

Nestlé Participants

Hugo Betz, *Nestlé Deutschland AG, Münich, Germany*

Laïla Dufour-Khouri, *Nestec Ltd., Vevey, Switzerland*

Helmut A. Grafinger, *Osterreische Nestlé Ges. mbH, Vienna, Austria*

Pierre R. Guesry, *Nestec Ltd., Vevey, Switzerland*

Hans-Jürgen Hoffmann, *Nestlé Deutschland AG, Münich, Germany*

Harald Lutz, *Nestlé Deutschland AG, Münich, Germany*

Nestlé Nutrition Workshop Series

Perinatology, edited by Erich Saling,
Nestlé Nutrition Workshop Series, Vol. 26,
Nestec, Ltd., Vevey/Raven Press, Ltd.,
New York © 1992.

Chorionic Villus Sampling throughout Gestation

Wolfgang Holzgreve and *P. Miny

*Department of Obstetrics and Gynecology and *Institute of Human Genetics,
Westfälische Wilhelms-Universität, Zentrum für Frauenheilkunde,
Albert-Schweitzer Strasse 33, D-4400 Münster, Germany*

Up to the spring of 1990 more than 60,000 chorionic villus samplings (CVS) in the first trimester (1) and more than 2,000 in the second and third trimesters (2) had been documented worldwide. Several single institutions reported first trimester series with more than 1,000 cases (3–7). Despite the still unsettled question of the safety of the procedure, CVS is currently being offered as an alternative to amniocentesis in many centers. It is obvious that CVS is the earliest and most rapid method available of obtaining cytogenetic, biochemical, and molecular genetic diagnoses. Since the mid 1980s second and third trimester CVS has also been developed as an alternative to fetal blood sampling for rapid prenatal diagnosis (8–11) with special benefits in pregnancies with abnormal amounts of amniotic fluid or when extremely fast results are required (12).

PATIENTS AND METHODS

In our Münster program, first trimester CVS was offered as an alternative to amniocentesis when patients registered in time and a diagnosis was feasible by this approach. From January 1, 1985, until December 31, 1989, 2,290 procedures were carried out in the first trimester and 301 procedures in the second and third trimesters (Table 1). The indications are summarized for the first trimester in Tables 2–4, for the second and third trimester in Table 5. For cytogenetic analysis our policy is to use metaphases from short-term incubation as well as cultured cells.

In the first trimester series, villi were aspirated transcervically under ultrasound guidance using a catheter with improved echogenicity as described previously (13) into RPMI medium with antibiotics. Transabdominal placentacentesis in the second and third trimester followed a protocol outlined by Holzgreve *et al.* (9) and Basaran *et al.* (10). Villi were separated immediately after the procedure under an inverted microscope. Maternal serum alpha-fetoprotein (AFP) was determined before and after sampling (14).

TABLE 1. *Chorionic villus sampling program, Münster 1985–1989*

Procedure	n
1st trimester transcervical	1,991
1st trimester transabdominal	299
2nd and 3rd trimester transabdominal	301
Total	2,591

In a few cases direct chromosome preparations were carried out on the same day. Villi were incubated routinely for 56 h in Chang's medium and processed essentially according to the method of Simoni *et al.* (15). We used colchicine (Merck, Darmstadt) for 3.5 h at a final concentration of 0.04 mg/ml and Carnoy's fixative in a 50% solution for 10 min followed by a 100% solution for a further 10 min. For the past 2 years slide preparation has been carried out by a device (ECT 85) purchased from E. J. Toulemonde, Paris.

Cultures were set up on cover slips in Leighton tubes after treatment of the villi with trypsin and collagenase according to Ledbetter (16).

RESULTS

Approximately 50% of all patients eligible for first trimester CVS chose amniocentesis after counseling, which included a detailed review of advantages and disadvantages of both procedures. First trimester CVS was performed in 16 twin pregnancies, four of which were mono- and 12 were dichorionic (Table 6). According to our experience with twin pregnancies (7) we recommend CVS in dichorionic pregnancies only when the two chorion frondosum sites can be clearly separated

TABLE 2. *Chorionic villus sampling program, Münster: 1st trimester, 1985–1989*

Indication	n	%
Maternal age	1,903	83.5
Previous child with chromosome anomaly	143	6.3
Risk for X-linked disease	55	2.4
Risk for metabolic disease	48	2.1
Risk for thalassemia or hemoglobinopathy	26	1.1
Parental balanced rearrangement	17	0.7
Suspicious ultrasound findings	3	0.1
Paternity test	2	—
Sex determination for campomelia diagnosis	2	—
Confirmation of aneuploidy	1	—
Others (e.g., "anxiety")	78	3.4
Total	2,278	99.6

TABLE 3. *Chorionic villus sampling program Münster, 1985–1989:*
autosomal recessive diseases

Indication	n	Examination
Cystic fibrosis	15	DNA
Pfaundler-Hurler disease	7	enzyme test
Sanfilippo III A disease	4	enzyme test
Adrenogenital syndrome	4	HLA, DNA
Krabbe's disease	4	enzyme test
Cystinosis	3	cystine determination
Gaucher's disease	2	enzyme test
Niemann-Pick disease	2	enzyme test
Zellweger syndrome	2	long chain fatty acids
Alpha-1-antitrypsin deficiency	1	DNA
Fructose intolerance	1	enzyme test
Tay-Sachs disease	1	enzyme test
GM_1 gangliosidosis	1	enzyme test
GM_2 gangliosidosis	1	enzyme test
Propionicacidemia	1	enzyme test
Total	49	

HLA, human leukocyte antigen.

TABLE 4. *Chorionic villus sampling program, Münster 1985–1989: X-linked diseases*

Indication	n	Examination
Duchenne muscular dystrophy	26	DNA
Hemophilia A	10	DNA
Hemophilia B	1	DNA
Menkes' syndrome	3	copper determination
Hunter's syndrome	3	enzyme test
Chorioideremia	2	DNA
X-linked hydrocephalus	2	sonography
Adrenoleukodystrophy	2	long chain fatty acids
Wiskott-Aldrich syndrome	2	PUBS
Norrie syndrome	2	DNA
X-linked thrombocytopenia	1	PUBS
Fragile X syndrome	1	DNA, chromosomes
Lowe syndrome	1	DNA
Incontinentia pigmenti	1	fetal skin biopsy
OTC deficiency	1	DNA, liver biopsy
Total	58	

PUBS, percutaneous umbilical blood sampling.
OTC, ornithine transcarbamylase deficiency.

TABLE 5. *Chorionic villus sampling program, Münster:*
2nd and 3rd trimesters, 1985–1989

Indication	n
Suspected rubella infection	3
Confirmation of aneuploidy	28
Late booking	50
Suspicious ultrasound findings	220
Total	301

sonographically. The rate of unsuccessful procedures due to insufficient amounts of tissue has dropped to 0.5% over the last 2 years (Fig. 1). In the first trimester we apply both the transcervical and transabdominal (Table 6) techniques depending on the individual characteristics of uterine and placental positions.

The outcome of pregnancies after first trimester CVS is summarized in Table 7. Due to a formalized protocol including phone interviews with the attending gynecologist and the mother, only four cases, who all had a normal ultrasound at 16 weeks, were lost to follow-up.

Second and third trimester CVS was performed transabdominally only. In three cases with maternal rubella infection during pregnancy placental biopsies were obtained in order to evaluate maternal-fetal transfer of the virus by cDNA testing of villi. Because West German law requires a 3-day waiting period between communication of the fetal diagnosis and termination of pregnancy we routinely offer confirmation of an abnormal result by placental biopsy within this period. In the third group (according to Table 5) rapid karyotyping was requested because the pregnancies were close to the 22 weeks postconception legal limit for terminations because of fetal disease. Most of the procedures were performed following the detection of suspicious ultrasound findings. The key finding in 38% of the cases (Table 8) was an abnormal amount of amniotic fluid. In this series placental biopsies were carried out after 12 completed postmenstrual weeks of pregnancy up to 41 weeks (Fig. 2) with peaks at 22/23 weeks (due to the legal limit mentioned above) and at 31/32 weeks (at the time of the second sonographic evaluation in the West German screening scheme).

TABLE 6. *Chorionic villus sampling program, Münster: 1st trimester, 1985–1989;*
number performed

Patients		Aspirations	
Singletons	2,262	Successful procedures	2,255
Twins monochorionic	4	Unsuccessful procedures	35
Twins dichorionic	12	Transcervical aspirations	1,991
Total	2,278	Transabdominal aspirations	299
		Total	2,290

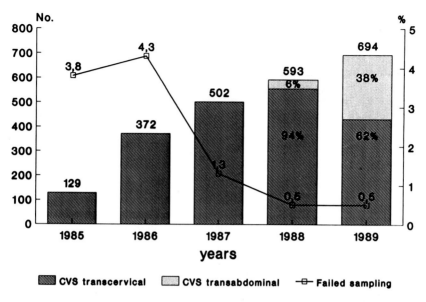

FIG. 1. Development of the chorionic villus sampling program in the first trimester of pregnancy at the University of Münster.

The cDNA testing for rubella allowed the diagnosis of fetal infection to be made as early as 14 weeks of pregnancy, which is considerably earlier than a diagnosis by fetal blood sampling at 23 weeks of gestation. In the second indication group (Table 5) all previous results were confirmed as expected with the exception of two cases with mosaicism in amniotic fluid cells. In these two cases placental biopsies were performed simultaneously with fetal blood sampling. In the second indication group rapid karyotyping revealed normal chromosome counts with the exception of a familial balanced reciprocal translocation, a *de novo*, presumably balanced, reciprocal translocation involving three chromosomes, and a trisomy 21. In this latter case an additional acrocentric had been seen in another laboratory but due to poor cell growth and technical quality, differentiation between a chromosome 21 and a Y chromosome had not been possible. We therefore performed "late CVS" at 23 weeks of pregnancy and confirmed trisomy 21. All pregnancies in indication group 1 (Table 5) were terminated with the exception of an X/XX mosaicism in amniotic

TABLE 7. *Chorionic villus sampling program, Münster: 1st trimester, 1985–1989*

	n	Failures	Therapeutic abortion	Continued pregnancy	Loss	Loss %	Deliveries
Transabdominal	299	—	7	292	8	2.7	124
Transcervical	1,991	35	70	1,921	94	4.9	1,807

TABLE 8. *Chorionic villus sampling program, Münster: 2nd and 3rd trimesters, 1985–1989; cytogenetic anomalies in presence of suspicious sonographic findings*

Key sonographic findings[a]	n	Cytogenetic anomalies	n
Oligo- or ahydramnios +/− IUGR	70	triploidy	5
		trisomy 21	1
		monosomy X	1
IUGR	24	trisomy 18	3
		triploidy	2
		trisomy 13	1
Hydrocephalus	14	46,XY/92,XXYY	1
NIHF	16	monosomy X	2
		47,XX, + 21/48,XX, + 18, + 21	1
Omphalocele	10	trisomy 18	3
		trisomy 13	1
		46,XY/49,XY, + 2, + 7, + 19	1
Polyhydramnios	16	trisomy 21	1
		trisomy 18	1
		trisomy 13	1
Hygroma colli	15	monosomy X	7
		trisomy 21	2
		trisomy 18	1
Hydronephrosis and/or dysplastic kidneys	16	trisomy 13	2
		trisomy 18	1
		46,XX/46,XX, + 9	1
Thoraco- and/or gastroschisis	4	trisomy 13	1
Partial mole	4	triploidy	2
Unilateral choroid plexus cyst	4	—	
Other abnormalities	31	trisomy 18	2
		trisomy 21	1
Total	224		45 (20%)

[a] Only the most obvious anomaly per case is listed. Usually there were several associated abnormalities detected by ultrasound.
IUGR, intrauterine growth retardation; NIHF, nonimmune hydrops fetalis.

fluid cells not confirmed in fetal blood or in trophoblastic tissue. All pregnancies in indication group 3 (Table 5) resulted in live births or at the time of writing were still ongoing uneventfully except the pregnancy with trisomy 21 in the fetus, and two pregnancies that were terminated for OTC deficiency and β-thalassemia, respectively.

All cytogenetic anomalies in group 4 (Table 5) are listed in Table 8 with reference to the key sonographic indication for karyotyping. The one case of trisomy 9 mosaicism was confirmed in amniotic fluid cells, and the + 21/ + 18, + 21 mosaicism by characteristic autopsy findings. The clinical significance of the two other mosaics is doubtful. Karyotyping was successful in all but three cases. There were no obvious short- or long-term complications associated with the placental biopsies such as hematomas or directly related intrauterine fetal demises. In the group of 45 cases with normal or balanced chromosome counts and normal ultrasound findings of indication group 2 there were no spontaneous abortions. However in the group of 180

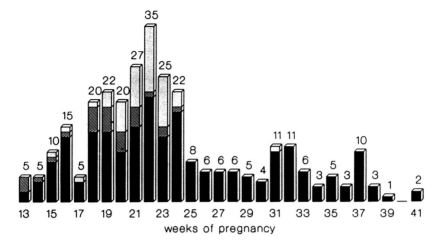

FIG. 2. Number of late CVS procedures (total 301 cases) per gestational week. *Black bars*, suspicious ultrasound findings; *hatched bars*, confirmation cases; *dotted bars*, late booking cases.

cases with suspicious ultrasound findings and normal karyotypes there were 16 intrauterine fetal demises, of which 13 were in association with severe oligohydramnios and/or intrauterine growth retardation and three with nonimmune hydrops fetalis (NIHF).

DISCUSSION

In our first trimester CVS series, aneuploidy (excluding unconfirmed mosaicism) interestingly enough does not seem to be significantly more frequent after CVS as compared to amniocentesis. An increased aneuploidy rate might be expected since CVS is carried out 5 to 6 weeks earlier than amniocentesis. Probably due to careful ultrasound examinations prior to CVS the number of "unnecessary" first trimester procedures in pregnancies prone to spontaneous abortion because of aneuploidy seems to be small. When compared to cytogenetic studies after amniocentesis (17,18) the frequency of true mosaicism and the risk of maternal cell contamination (MCC) is clearly increased after CVS.

In contrast to DNA studies from chorionic villi (19,20), maternal cell contamination is still of some concern in cytogenetic as well as in biochemical studies. From our own experience the frequency of MCC is clearly correlated with the expertise in handling the biopsy specimen.

In view of the reported false-negative diagnoses from direct preparations, we recommend the simultaneous use of both direct preparation and cultured cells in routine cytogenetic diagnosis from chorionic tissue. With the exception of two cases all false negatives observed so far occurred after direct preparation, whereas cultured cells gave a correct result (7). The frequency of false negatives has been estimated as approximately 1 in 1,000 (21). We encountered two cases among a total of 2,591 cytogenetic diagnoses.

Mosaicism not only accounts for the majority of false-negative findings but also for most of the false positives. There have been only a few instances of apparently nonmosaic false positives (22–24) but there are numerous reports of mosaics detected at a rate of around 1% in most large series (5,23). The embryological background has been elucidated by Kalousek and coworkers (25–27) and Crane and Cheung (28), who considered that cultured chorionic cells were more likely to represent the fetal chromosome complement. At present we recommend that amniocentesis should be offered in all cases of mosaicism, whether diagnosed after direct preparation or in cultured cells exclusively, or by both methods. Accumulation of more data on mosaicism in chorionic villi may help to differentiate between high- and low-risk situations in the near future. At present, a substantial proportion of women undergoing CVS will have to accept the risk of an additional procedure for the sake of reassurance when mosaicism is diagnosed, even if the confirmation rate at amniocentesis seems to be low.

By combined application of culture techniques and direct preparation as well as by consideration of such safeguards as careful separation of biopsies and amniocentesis in all doubtful cases, the overall frequency of diagnostic errors in first trimester CVS is not different from that in published amniocentesis series. The obvious advantages of this early and fast procedure are not counterbalanced by a reduced validity of the cytogenetic diagnosis.

Because chorionic villi are a rich source of DNA and molecular genetic as well as biochemical diagnoses are very reliable, we find first trimester CVS especially beneficial in pregnancies at risk for autosomal recessive and X-linked diseases.

Our series of transabdominal procedures in the first trimester is too small to allow a meaningful comparison to the transcervical route. However, two controlled studies, one of them randomized, did not reveal a significant difference in loss rates after CVS as compared to amniocentesis (29,30).

The cytogenetic techniques, namely direct chromosome preparation, can also be successfully applied after placentacentesis in the second and third trimester. When the procedure was carried out following the sonographic diagnosis of fetal abnormalities the rate of chromosomal anomalies was as high as 20%. This approach offers an alternative to fetal blood sampling for rapid karyotyping especially in high-risk cases with oligo- or polyhydramnios.

SUMMARY

More than 60,000 first trimester chorionic villus samplings (CVS) performed up to the spring of 1990 document that this fairly new procedure can already be considered as an established alternative to amniocentesis worldwide. More than 2,000 placental biopsies taken in the second and third trimester for rapid prenatal diagnosis show that this more recent alternative to fetal blood sampling is gaining popularity.

Up to the end of 1989, 2,290 first trimester procedures and 301 late chorionic villus samplings had been performed in Münster. In the first trimester the rate of pregnancy terminations was not significantly different from that in our amniocentesis program. We use both transcervical and transabdominal techniques depending on the individual uterine and placental positions. In the second and third trimester all procedures are transabdominal. The main indications for late CVS were late booking, confirmation of abnormal results, cDNA testing for rubella, and suspicious ultrasound findings. In the latter group the rate of chromosomal abnormalities was 20%. Two recent large scale studies have shown that the procedure-related complication rate of early CVS is not significantly different from amniocentesis and the same seems to apply for late CVS.

ACKNOWLEDGMENT

This research is supported by grants from "Bundesminister für Forschung and Technologie."

REFERENCES

1. Jackson LG. *CVS Newsletter*, January, 1990.
2. Holzgreve W, Miny P, Gerlach B, Westendorp A, Ahlert D, Horst J. Benefits of placental biopsies for rapid karyotyping in the second and third trimester (late CVS) in high risk pregnancies. *Am J Obstet Gynecol* 1990;162:1188–92.
3. Simoni G, Gimelli G, Cuoco C, et al. First trimester fetal karyotyping: one thousand diagnoses. *Hum Genet* 1986;72:203–9.
4. Jackson LG, Wapner RA, Barr MA. Safety of chorionic villus sampling. *Lancet* 1986;1:674.
5. Hogge WA, Schonberg SA, Golbus MS. Chorionic villus sampling: experience of the first 1000 cases. *Am J Obstet Gynecol* 1986;154:1249–52.
6. Sachs E, Jahoda MGJ, Kleijer WJ, Pijpers L, Galjaard H. Impact of first-trimester chromosome, DNA, and metabolic studies on pregnancies at high genetic risk: experience with 1000 cases. *Am J Med Genet* 1988;29:293–303.
7. Miny P, Basaran S, Pawlowitzki IH, et al. Validity of cytogenetic analyses from trophoblast tissue throughout gestation. *Am J Med Genet* 1989;33:136–41.
8. Nicolaides KH, Soothill PW, Rodeck CH, Warren RC. Why confine chorionic villus (placental) biopsy to the first trimester? *Lancet* 1986;1:543–4.
9. Holzgreve W, Miny P, Basaran S, Fuhrmann W, Beller FK. Safety of placental biopsy in the second and third trimesters. *N Engl J Med* 1987;317:1159.
10. Basaran S, Miny P, Pawlowitzki IH, Horst J, Holzgreve W. Rapid karyotyping for prenatal diagnosis in the second and third trimesters of pregnancy. *Prenat Diagn* 1988;8:315–20.
11. Monni G, Ibba RM, Olla G, Rossatelli C, Cao A. Prenatal diagnosis of β-thalassemia by second trimester chorionic villus sampling. *Prenat Diagn* 1988;8:447–51.
12. Holzgreve W, Miny P, Schloo R. "Late CVS" international registry compilation of data from 24 centers. *Prenat Diagn* 1990;10:159–67.
13. Holzgreve W, Miny P. Chorionic villi sampling with an echogenic catheter: experiences with the first 500 cases. *J Perinat Med* 1987;15:244–9.
14. Fuhrmann W, Altland K, Köhler A, et al. Feto-maternal transfusion after chorionic villus sampling. *Hum Genet* 1988;78:83–5.
15. Simoni G, Brambati B, Danesino C, et al. Efficient direct chromosome analysis and enzyme determinations from chorionic villi samples in the first trimester of pregnancy. *Hum Genet* 1983;63:349–57.
16. Ledbetter S. Quoted in Jackson L, *CVS Newsletter*, August 26, 1984.

17. Loft A, Tabor A. Discordance between prenatal cytogenetic diagnosis and outcome of pregnancy. *Prenat Diagn* 1984;4:51–9.
18. Hsu LYF. Prenatal diagnosis of chromosome abnormalities. In: Milunsky A, ed. *Genetic disorders and the fetus*. London: Plenum Press. 1986;115–83.
19. De Martinville B, Blakemore K, Mahoney MJ, Francke U. DNA-analysis of first trimester chorionic villus biopsies: test for maternal contamination. *Am J Hum Genet* 1984;36:1357–68.
20. Oehme R, Jonatha WD, Horst J. DNA-diagnosis of sickle cell anemia from chorionic villi: possible influence of maternal cell contamination. *Hum Genet* 1986;73:186–7.
21. Simoni G, Fraccaro M, Gimelli G, Maggi F, Dagna Bricarelli F. False-positive and false-negative findings on chorionic villus sampling. *Prenat Diagn* 1987;7:671–2.
22. Simoni G, Gimelli G, Cuoco C, et al. Discordance between prenatal cytogenetic diagnosis after chorionic villus sampling and chromosomal constitution of the fetus. In: Fraccaro M, Simoni G, Brambati B, eds. First trimester fetal diagnosis. Berlin: Springer-Verlag, 1985;137–43.
23. Mikkelsen M, Ayme S. Chromosomal findings in chorionic villi: a collaborative study. In: Vogel F, Sperling K, eds. *Human genetics*. New York: Springer-Verlag, 1987;597–605.
24. Green JE, Dorfman A, Jones SL, Bender S, Patten L, Schulman JD. Chorionic villus sampling: experience with an initial 940 cases. *Obstet Gynecol* 1988;71:208–12.
25. Kalousek DK, Dill FJ. Chromosomal mosaicism confined to the placenta in human conceptions. *Science* 1983;221:665–7.
26. Kalousek DK. Mosaicism confined to chorionic tissue in human gestations. In: Fracaro M, Simoni G, Brambati B, eds. First trimester fetal diagnosis. Berlin: Springer Verlag, 1985;136.
27. Kalousek DK, Dill FJ, Pantzar T, McGillivray TC, Yong SL, Wilson RD. Confined chorionic mosaicism in prenatal diagnosis. *Hum Genet* 1987;77:163–7.
28. Crane JP, Cheung SW. An embryogenic model to explain cytogenetic inconsistencies observed in chorionic villus versus fetal tissue. *Prenat Diagn* 1988;8:119–29.
29. Rhoads GG, Jackson LG, Schlesselman SI, et al. The safety and efficacy of chorionic villus sampling for early prenatal diagnosis and cytogenetic abnormalities. *N Engl J Med* 1989;320:609–17.
30. Canadian Collaborative CVS-Amniocentesis Clinical Trial Group. Multicenter randomized clinical trial of chorionic villus sampling and amniocentesis. *Lancet* 1989;1:1–7.

DISCUSSION

Dr. Van Geijn: How often do you obtain false-positive results with placental biopsies, particularly mosaicism? And how often do you fail to obtain actively mitotic cells in the second and third trimesters? Supporters of cordocentesis claim that these problems are less with that technique. How successful have you been in karyotyping placental biopsies in the third trimester?

Dr. Holzgreve: In our reported experiences with 1,184 first trimester chorion villus samplings (CVS) we did not find any nonmosaic false-positive results, using direct preparation and chorion villus culture simultaneously. We considered that we had identified "true mosaicism" when two or more aneuploid cells were observed after direct preparation or when aneuploidy was present in different culture vessels or in at least two different colonies on one slide. Among the first 1,184 cases, 15 such instances were diagnosed, of which only two were confirmed in amniotic fluid cell culture. The remaining 13 may be considered as false-positive (1.1%). Placentae were available at term in six of these cases and placental mosaicism was confirmed in all. All 13 pregnancies went to term and the mean birth weight was 3,683 g. We presently recommend amniocentesis after first trimester CVS or cordocentesis after second trimester CVS in all cases of mosaicism.

Regarding late rapid karyotyping, in our series of 301 placental biopsies in the second and third trimesters we have been able to obtain a karyotype from direct preparations in all but four cases on the first attempt. Therefore, in almost all cases with ultrasonographic anomalies where rapid karyotyping is required for decision making, we think action is justified on the basis of the direct preparations without waiting for culture results.

Dr. Guesry: In view of the enormous current expense of health care and the temptation to limit the use of such highly sophisticated procedures, do you have any cost-benefit analyses?

Dr. Holzgreve: We have not done cost-benefit analyses ourselves. It is obvious, however, from previous calculations of this kind, that all established methods of prenatal diagnosis are cost-effective, through the prevention of unnecessary obstetric intervention, long-term care of handicap, and so on. Monni and Cao in Cagliari have shown that late CVS with direct DNA extraction is much more effective and practicable in diagnosing thalassemia than even the established second trimester amniocentesis.

Dr. Marini: I don't completely agree about this work in Sardinia since with bone marrow transplantation life expectancy is now rather good for thalassemia. Of course the parents must be given the opportunity for prenatal diagnosis but the problem is to give the best genetic advice. It is very important to explain to the parents all the possibilities of therapy.

Dr. Golbus: We have found that many patients who chose not to have amniocentesis when it was the only technique available because the answer came too late were willing to have antenatal diagnosis when chorionic villus sampling became available. We also found that in both autosomal and sex chromosome anomalies, couples who chose CVS had their answer earlier and were more likely to choose termination of pregnancy than couples who had elected for amniocentesis.

Dr. Holzgreve: It is our experience that couples who seek prenatal diagnosis often already have an affected child who is well integrated into their families and taken care of in a most impressive way. They might then select prenatal diagnosis because they don't want to have another child with the same handicaps. I feel it would be arrogant of a physician to tell them that they were doing one thing excellently but that the other was unacceptable. Unfortunately the media have a tendency to create artificial conflicts between caring for handicap and prenatal diagnosis.

As far as thalassemia is concerned, clearly the issue of bone marrow transplantation needs to be discussed at length with the parents, but the successes reported so far are still limited and long-term results are not completely clear yet.

Dr. Golbus: On another matter, it is important to remember that, when comparing fetal loss following transabdominal and transcervical procedures, most publications have quoted *total* transcervical rates—i.e., the transcervical losses both before transabdominal CVS was available and after it was available. These need to be broken down, because the most important factor associated with fetal loss is a difficult procedure. For example a fundal placenta, a small amount of villi, and more than one insertion, all represent difficult procedures. These are situations where today a transabdominal route would be chosen, and they then become easy procedures. In studies which have taken this into account, including our own, no difference in loss rate has been shown between transcervical and transabdominal procedures.

Dr. Saling: Is there any information about the frequency of infection caused by the transvaginal method?

Dr. Holzgreve: In the United States National Institutes of Health controlled trial, no septic shock was reported in more than 4,000 women investigated. The rate of less serious infections was around 12% which is probably not different from that expected in women with spontaneous abortions without previous interventions. Proper technical precautions minimize the risks of infection, particularly the atraumatic direct insertion of the catheter through the cervix and the proper disinfection of the exterior of the cervix.

Dr. Golbus: One of the simplest and most important preventive measures is to change the catheter for a fresh one after each unsuccessful pass.

Dr. Saling: One of the main reasons for infection following transabdominal CVS is that the skin is not disinfected sufficiently, and particularly that the disinfecting solution has not been given enough time to act. Since we have appreciated this we have had extremely low infection rates by this route.

Dr. Holzgreve: It is worth recalling that no prenatal intervention is without risk and therefore a proper indication should always be present.

Dr. Guesry: It seems that in Germany there was a sharp increase in early pregnancy terminations after the Chernobyl accident. Was CVS able to make the distinction between justified and unjustified fear of malformation?

Dr. Holzgreve: A very careful study coordinated by Professor Sperling from Berlin showed that there was no evidence for an increase in cytogenetic abnormalities related to the Chernobyl nuclear accident. We therefore did not consider this as an indication for a prenatal procedure and there is no clear evidence that the rate of terminations in Germany went up considerably because of Chernobyl.

Dr. Saling: I should like to make the recommendation that when we refer to fetal blood sampling in the field of antenatal diagnosis, we should call it "antepartum fetal blood sampling" to avoid confusion with intrapartum fetal scalp blood sampling.

Dr. Holzgreve: This is a very appropriate recommendation since there is no agreed terminology. Some prefer the term "cordocentesis" and the Americans have introduced the acronym "PUBS" (percutaneous umbilical blood sampling). I prefer "antepartum fetal blood sampling" because we do not necessarily only get blood from the cord.

Dr. Freye: What about the results of early amniocentesis?

Dr. Holzgreve: I am somewhat critical about the results of so-called early amniocentesis procedures reported so far. They commonly include cases performed at 14 to 15 weeks gestation, at which time the result would not be available in the first trimester at a time when termination could be performed by D & C. There have been only a few cases reported of amniocentesis at 8 to 9 weeks, when CVS is already possible. The rate of loss seems clearly higher with amniocentesis at this gestational age and there are additional problems including tenting of the membranes, equivocal acetylcholinesterase findings, and worries about the relatively large volume of fluid withdrawn in comparison to later amniocentesis. Therefore I don't think early amniocentesis is a real competitor for first trimester CVS yet.

Perinatology, edited by Erich Saling,
Nestlé Nutrition Workshop Series, Vol. 26,
Nestec, Ltd., Vevey/Raven Press, Ltd.,
New York © 1992.

Modern Methods of DNA Diagnosis

Karl-Heinz Grzeschik

*Abteilung für Allgemeine Humangenetik, Medizinisches Zentrum für Humangenetik
der Universität Marburg, Bahnhofstrasse 7A, D-3550 Marburg, Germany*

Progress in molecular biology and biotechnology has created promising possibilities for the analysis at the DNA level of basic defects underlying many genetic diseases. The new achievements in finding the specific position of genes in the human genome, in dissecting their structure, reading their base sequence, and in understanding the biochemical mechanisms of their function and, eventually, malfunction lead to profound new insights into the pathology of inherited diseases.

In clinical practice this progress has not only led to new approaches in pre- or postnatal diagnosis, but in specific situations it has enabled predictions about the phenotypic severity to be made and, even more important, it has given new hope for the design of novel treatments.

The progress made so far mainly relates to the analysis of disorders due to a defect in a single gene. Therefore approaches to the diagnosis of clinically relevant mutations in genes resulting in genetic diseases with a clear Mendelian inheritance of a characteristic phenotype, either autosomal dominant, autosomal recessive, or X-linked, will be discussed.

THE GENETIC MAP IS THE BASIS FOR DIAGNOSIS

The prerequisite for unequivocal diagnosis of a genetic defect is the description of nucleic acid sequences that are informative in that disease. This goal of finding the gene sequence has been achieved for an impressive list of disorders caused by defects on all human chromosomes and the mitochondrial genome (1). However, given the huge number (approximately 5×10^4) of genes encoded by approximately 3–5% of the total 3×10^9 base pairs distributed along the 24 different human chromosomes, a major effort will be necessary until all human genes are identified. We have the privilege of working in this field in the exciting period during which the goal of a complete genetic map of our species is no longer a fantastic vision but one that will probably be achieved within the next decade.

As soon as the gene causing a disease is identified, the underlying changes of the genetic information at this chromosomal site can be analyzed in patients, and the pathophysiology of the disease can be related to the malfunctioning or missing gene

PROBE

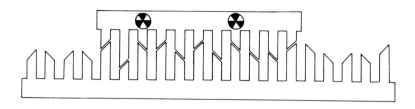

TEMPLATE

FIG. 1. Molecular hybridization. A single stranded molecular *probe* recognizes its complementary template sequences among millions of other fragments. The binding is monitored with labels incorporated in the probe stand. Reporter groups used for labeling of nucleic acid probes can be radioisotopes like ^{3}H, ^{32}P, ^{35}S, enzymes like peroxidase or alkaline phosphatase, fluorophores, or chelated rare earth metal ions (3). The detection procedures accordingly vary from autoradiography to scintillation counting, gamma ray spectometry, colorimetry, fluorimetry, and luminimetry.

product. In addition to the most extensively studied hemoglobinopathies and thalassemias, many of the more frequent genetic disorders like cystic fibrosis, alpha-1-antitrypsin deficiency, hemophilias A and B and the other disorders of the coagulation cascade, and Duchenne and Becker type muscular dystrophies, have been characterized at the gene level, as have disorders of collagen, inborn errors of amino acid metabolism, endocrine disorders, lysosomal storage diseases, and genes related to the appearance of familial tumors like retinoblastoma (2,3).

RAPID TECHNICAL PROGRESS TOWARD FAST AND
RELIABLE DIAGNOSIS

The discovery of gene sequences informative for specific disorders has been accompanied by the rapid development of methods that allow us to monitor these sequences pre- or postnatally in individual probands.

The material to be tested is mainly DNA, which can be extracted from all nucleated tissues and cells, e.g., peripheral lymphocytes, biopsy specimens, amniotic fluid cells, or chorionic villi. Analyzing a specific sequence in a sample of genomic DNA means searching for a few hundred base pairs on the background of about 6×10^9 base pairs contained in each diploid nucleus. The procedure sensitive enough to trace this small piece of information is called DNA or RNA hybridization (Fig. 1). A labeled *probe*, a copy of the sequence to be searched, binds to the genome *template* if it is identical to the original, and does not bind strongly if the two text fragments differ by even a single letter. If total genomic DNA is to be analyzed in this way, typically 5 to 20 μg contained in about 10^6 nucleated cells are required for each test,

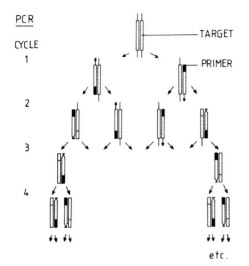

FIG. 2. Polymerase chain reaction (PCR). The PCR is an enzymatic method of synthesizing millions of copies of a discrete DNA or RNA fragment. Its use requires the synthesis of two flanking oligonucleotide primers that hybridize to opposite strands of the target sequence. The primers are oriented with their 3' ends pointing toward each other. The template is denatured by heat. Then the primers anneal to their complementary sequences. Polymerase subsequently extends the primers. During repeated cycles of this procedure the sequence defined by the 5' ends of the PCR primers is amplified predominantly (4–6).

to obtain a detectable hybridization signal with a radiolabeled probe. This limits the number of analyses available from small samples, such as for instance the material obtained by chorion villus sampling at the 10th week of pregnancy or by an amniocentesis performed in the 16th week.

This limitation can be overcome by a brilliant method called polymerase chain reaction (PCR) developed in 1985 (Fig. 2) (4–6). Discrete short DNA or RNA sequences (targets) can be amplified exponentially to a 10^6- to 10^7-fold increase in copy number within hours and are then easily amenable to the various approaches to genome analysis for rapid prenatal diagnosis and carrier testing for inherited disorders. The source DNA can originate from a single human oocyte which allows the option of preimplantation diagnosis of inherited disease (7). The PCR technology lends itself to automation, and the development of diagnostic equipment based on the use of PCR and various types of hybridization assays is proceeding fast (3).

Each mutated gene can differ from the normal allele in single nucleotide pairs as well as through changes such as deletions, insertions, duplications, and translocations of DNA segments; such changes can cover a wide size range from a few base pairs to gross events that can be detected under the light microscope as cytogenetic peculiarities. This broad spectrum of changes is monitored routinely with three basic technical approaches: (a) comparison of DNA fragment lengths after digestion with a restriction enzyme and electrophoretic separation (RFLP) (8,9); (b) allele-specific hybridization with oligonucleotides (ASO) (10); and (c) allele-specific amplification (ASA) (11) by PCR (Fig. 3).

PCR even provides material for direct sequence analysis of a gene region from individual probands. Sequencing, however, has not been widely used so far in routine diagnostics, nor have procedures like oligonucleotide ligation, RNase A technique, and denaturing gradient gel electrophoresis, which are capable of analyzing point mutations (3).

FIG. 3. Procedures for the diagnosis of mutations in the human genome. (A) RFL analysis: lengths or presence of restriction fragments as indication of a mutation. Restriction endonuclease analysis of DNA can detect mutations within a recognition site of the enzyme, absence of a gene or part of a gene, as well as the presence of abnormal DNA fragments in the rearranged part of a gene. Fragments obtained by enzyme action on PCR products can be visualized by direct staining after size fractionation by gel electrophoresis. Genomic DNA is analyzed by the Southern blot procedure: after cleavage and electrophoretic separation the fragments are rendered single stranded, transferred to filters, and hybridized with a single-stranded labeled molecular probe (8). Polymorphic variation within a specific DNA sequence of different homologous chromosomes is detected as restriction fragment length polymorphism (RFLP) (9). Combination of RFLP alleles at neighboring loci on the chromosome are called "haplotypes." (B) Hybridiza-

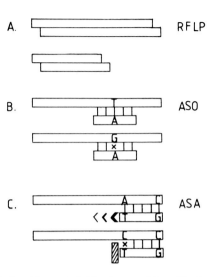

tion with an allele-specific oligonucleotide (ASO). Under stringent hybridization conditions (3), oligonucleotides bind firmly only to templates without base pair mismatches. A point mutation within the template can be detected with the appropriate synthetic oligonucleotide. (C) Allele-specific amplification. A target DNA is amplified only in the PCR reaction if the 3'-ends of the extension primers show the base homologous to the target base at this position (11). Mismatches due to a mutation in the target sequence at this position are detected by lack of the appropriate PCR product.

DIRECT AND INDIRECT DIAGNOSIS OF GENETIC DISEASES

In only very few monogenic diseases is the same base pair altered in all patients. The best studied example is sickle cell anemia where a point mutation exchanges one amino acid of the β-globin chain. A low mutation rate and functional restraints within the affected molecule may be responsible for this exception. For several diseases a limited number of mutations is detected in the majority of patients from a particular population. β-Thalassemia, alpha-1-antitrypsin deficiency, phenylketonuria, and cystic fibrosis belong to this category, and are caused predominantly by single or few nucleotide differences (2). In many cases, unfortunately, individual persons or families carry their "private" mutations with the result that for autosomal diseases many patients may be compound heterozygotes.

This widespread diversity of the mutations in individual genetic diseases prohibits the development of simply designed large-scale screening in the general population. Only when the sequence defect to be expected in a given proband can be predicted with a high degree of certainty can a *direct diagnosis* of this sequence give a clear-cut yes or no answer.

If this knowledge is not available, due to heterogeneity at the gene level or because the gene has not yet been found or studied well enough, an *indirect diagnosis* may at best delineate a probability for the presence of the mutated gene (see Example

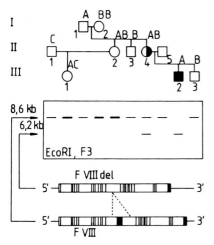

FIG. 4. A family with deletion in the F VIII-gene causing hemophilia A. The factor VIII-gene is shown at the *bottom*. F VIII del depicts the deleted gene. The autoradiogram is shown in the *middle*, the pedigree on *top*. The DNA samples in each lane of the autoradiogram are from the persons in the pedigree straight above the lane. Letters A, B, C in the pedigree represent haplotypes defined by different polymorphic markers associated with the factor VIII-gene in each subject.

1). In practice both approaches must be available in a diagnostic unit and indirect diagnosis should be applied when direct approaches fail in a given case.

The procedure will be outlined using three cases of frequent genetic diseases with different types of mutations.

EXAMPLE 1. Case of a family of a boy with hemophilia A, who requested genetic counseling (Fig. 4).

First the chromosome carrying the mutation was identified by indirect gene diagnosis. Characteristic polymorphic sites (Fig. 3A) close to and within the gene were used to mark the X chromosome with the mutant F VIII gene. The combination of specific RFLP alleles seen on the chromosome is called "haplotype" A. Starting from the index patient the segregation of this chromosome throughout the family can be monitored. Due to a physical and genetic distance between the F VIII gene and one of the markers on the chromosome there is an error rate for each prediction of about 1% to 5%.

The affected boy shared his haplotype (chromosome) with several family members including an unaffected uncle and his unaffected maternal grandfather. The mutation could have occurred in his mother or his grandfather.

Since 4–5% of hemophilia patients show intragenic deletions (2) a series of F VIII cDNA probes was used to search for deletions in the patient's DNA. A deletion eliminating intron 14 was detected. Direct diagnosis of the mutation was then possible using a probe from intron 14 next to one of the break points of the deletions. Indicative of the deleted gene was a 6.2 kb Eco RI fragment. Since this fragment was already present in the patient's mother, the mutation obviously occurred in the maternal grandfather. A carrier status for II, 2 and III, 1 was excluded. Prenatal diagnosis was carried out during a subsequent pregnancy. The boy III, 3 was shown to be unaffected both by haplotype and by direct analysis. The study extended over a long period of time, and this would have been too long for immediate prenatal

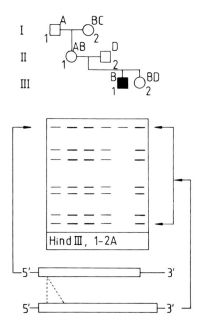

FIG. 5. A family with deletion in the dystrophin gene causing Duchenne muscular dystrophy (DMD). The normal and the deleted gene are depicted diagrammatically at the *bottom*. The autoradiogram is shown in the *middle*. Individuals with the intact gene show seven bands, the patient with the deletion only one. The pedigree is shown on *top*. Letters above the symbols in the pedigree represent haplotypes defined by different polymorphic markers associated with the dystrophin genes of each subject. Lanes on the autoradiogram correlate to the persons indicated above the lane in the pedigree.

diagnosis. This stresses the need for organized cooperation on the part of a family requesting genetic counseling and advice in family planning.

EXAMPLE 2. Case of the younger sister of a patient suffering from Duchenne muscular dystrophy (DMD) who was shown by haplotype analysis to have inherited from her mother the same haplotype on the X chromosome as her brother (Fig. 5).

Since more than 50% of all mutations in DMD are caused by deletions of the exceptionally long dystrophin gene, cDNA probes were used to screen for such an event (12–14) in the patient's DNA, and probe cDNA 1–2A on a genomic HindIII blot indeed indicated the loss of a series of restriction fragments. Dosage analysis suggested that neither the patient's sister nor his mother were heterozygous. This type of carrier diagnosis, in contrast to the unequivocal result in affected fetuses, suffers from a risk of misdiagnosis of about 5% (13). Strategies to overcome this limitation involve the search for deletion break points with intron probes (13) and discrimination of the homologous gene segments with polymorphic restriction sites.

EXAMPLE 3. Case of a family with a son suffering from cystic fibrosis (CF) (Fig. 6) who was tested for RFLP alleles marking the parental chromosomes carrying the defect. In both parents the CF mutation occurred on the background of haplotype B. This haplotype in the German population is found in about 84% of CF chromosomes (15). Due to the high linkage disequilibrium between B and CF it was likely that the mother's sister (II, 4) was a carrier as well. Her husband also happened to have haplotype B on one of his chromosomes. Since B is quite frequent in the North

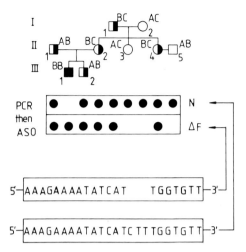

FIG. 6. A family with cystic fibrosis (CF). The mutation responsible for CF in this family and a normal allele are indicated in the oligonucleotide sequence at the *bottom*. The result of hybridization with allele-specific oligonucleotides is shown in the *middle*, the pedigree on *top*. All persons in the pedigree were tested for the presence of both alleles. The letters in the pedigree represent haplotypes defined by different polymorphic markers associated with the CF gene in each subject.

European population without a CF mutation (about 15%) (16) a clear answer could not be given.

Since the CF gene was detected in the meantime (17–19) the family's DNA was retyped with a procedure based on ASO analysis of a segment amplified by PCR that included the expected site of the mutation, a three nucleotide deletion, Delta F508. All persons carrying the deletion could be identified.

The husband, II, 5, did not show the Delta F deletion. However, since about 23% of CF chromosomes must have the mutation elsewhere in the gene (20) an unequivocal answer as to whether or not he is heterozygous still cannot be given. Due to this uncertainty a general screening procedure for CF is not yet available.

PROSPECTS

The sequence of diagnostic steps outlined in the three cases described above is obviously not optimal with regard to efficiency and limitation of costs, but rather reflects the continuing improvement of diagnostic systems with increasing knowledge about individual genes. It should be clear, even from these few examples, that the end point of this development has by no means been reached as yet.

Even in the well-studied genetic diseases discussed here, unequivocal answers to diagnostic questions cannot be given for all situations, and in some cases diagnosis in a single family involves a degree of effort comparable to that required for a research project. Unless further brilliant and surprising technical developments such as the invention of PCR dramatically change the outlook, the ultimate relief from the burden imposed by the great variety of possible mutations at many gene loci may be provided by automated high-speed sequencing and computer programs, able to analyze the functional efficiency of the gene product for individual probands via the gene sequences observed. It is hoped the genome mapping and sequencing project mentioned above will provide the impetus for the development of these high-technology diagnostic tools.

REFERENCES

1. Kidd KK, Klinger HP, Ruddle FH, eds. Human Gene Mapping 10: Tenth international workshop on human gene mapping. *Cytogenet Cell Genet* 1989;51:1–1148.
2. Antonarakis SE. Diagnosis of genetic disorders at the DNA level. *N Engl J Med* 1989;320:153–69.
3. Landegren U, Kaiser R, Caskey CT, Hood L. DNA-diagnostics—molecular techniques and automation. *Science* 1988;242:229–37.
4. Saiki RK, Scharf S, Faloona F, *et al*. Enzymatic amplification of β-globin genomic sequences and restriction site analysis for diagnosis of sickle cell anemia. *Science* 1985;230:1350–4.
5. White TJ, Arnheim N, Erlich HA. The polymerase chain reaction. *TIG* 1989;5:185–9.
6. Boehm CD. Use of polymerase chain reaction for diagnosis of inherited disorders. *Clin Chem* 1989;35:1843–8.
7. Coutelle C, Williams C, Handyside A, Hardy K, Winston R, Williamson R. Genetic analysis of DNA from single human oocytes: a model for preimplantation diagnosis of cystic fibrosis. *Br Med J* 1989;299:22–4.
8. Southern EM. Gel electrophoresis of restriction fragments. *Methods Enzymol* 1979;68:152–76.
9. Kan YW, Dozy AM. Polymorphism of DNA sequence adjacent to human β-globin structural gene. Relationship to sickle cell mutation. *Proc Natl Acad Sci USA* 1978;75:5631–5.
10. Engelke DR, Hoener PA, Collins FS. Direct sequencing of enzymatically amplified human genomic DNA. *Proc Natl Acad Sci USA* 1988;85:544–8.
11. Okayama H, Curiel DT, Branthy ML, Holmes MD, Crystal KG. Rapid, nonradioactive detection of mutations in the human genome by allele-specific amplification. *J Lab Clin Med* 1989;114:105–13.
12. Koenig M, Hoffmann EP, Bertelson CJ, Monaco AP, Teener C, Kunkel LM. Complete cloning of the Duchenne muscular dystrophy (DMD) cDNA and preliminary genomic organization of the DMD gene in normal and affected individuals. *Cell* 1987;50:509–17.
13. Speer A, Spiegler AWJ, Hanke R, *et al*. Possibilities and limitation of prenatal diagnosis and carrier determination for Duchenne and Becker muscular dystrophy using cDNA probes. *J Med Genet* 1989;26:1–5.
14. Passos-Bueno MR, Rapaport D, Love D, *et al*. Screening of deletions in the dystrophin gene with the cDNA probes Cf23a, Cf56a and Cf115. *J Med Genet* 1990;27:145–50.
15. Weber J, Aulehla-Scholz C, Kaiser R, *et al*. Cystic fibrosis: typing 89 German families with linked DNA probes. *Hum Genet* 1988;81:54–6.
16. Lemna WK, Feldman GL, Kerem B-S, *et al*. Mutation analysis for heterozygote detection and the prenatal diagnosis of cystic fibrosis. *N Engl J Med* 1990;322:291–6.
17. Kerem B-S, Rommens JM, Buchanan JA, *et al*. Identification of the cystic fibrosis gene: genetic analysis. *Science* 1989;245:1073–80.
18. Riordan JR, Rommens JM, Kerem B-S, *et al*. Identification of the cystic fibrosis gene: cloning and characterization of complementary DNA. *Science* 1989;245:1066–73.
19. Rommens JM, Iannuzi MC, Kerem B-S, *et al*. Identification of the cystic fibrosis gene: chromosome walking and jumping. *Science* 1989;245:1059–65.
20. Reis A, Bremer S, Schlösser M, *et al*. Distribution pattern of the delta F508 mutation in the CFTR gene on CF linked marker haplotypes in the German population (abstract). 2. Tagung der Gesellschaft für Humangenetik, Bonn, 28–31 March, 1990; 223.

DISCUSSION

Dr. Van Geijn: In prenatal diagnosis, we are always on the lookout for techniques that provide answers as early as possible, as correctly as possible, and give the maximum information. I have the feeling that we aren't making full use of the available possibilities, particularly with regard to DNA diagnosis. What is the future of DNA studies in the diagnosis of trisomies?

Dr. Grzeschik: Quick diagnosis of sex can already be done. For trisomies one needs a very detailed map. For trisomy 21 you have to know exactly which minimum sequence is the one that causes trisomy. The presence of this sequence could be determined by one of the approaches described, probably the PCR technique. But this would mean a sort of quantification using the PCR technique, which is not easy. So the first step is to improve the map so that eventually, if one knows which regions one is looking for, it may be possible to apply cytogenetic techniques to replace light microscopic analysis of banded chromosomes.

Dr. Golbus: In our laboratory we are using chromosome-specific probes—ones that recognize only number 21 for example. We use *in situ* hybridization, which means that we can look at each specific cell. One advantage is that you don't need a metaphase cell; an interphase cell is sufficient. You simply hybridize with a fluorescent 21-specific probe and count the number of fluorescent dots, either two or three. We have developed this to the point where we can analyze the cells from 2 to 3 ml of amniotic fluid as a 24-hour procedure. I think this technique has more promise than PCR and densitometry because of the problem of recognizing three *versus* two with the latter.

Dr. Grzeschik: We run into the same problem with hybridization on Southern blots when the fragments are small. It depends on if the system is sensitive enough to detect triple doses of chromosome 21 fragments.

Dr. Golbus: The probes being used are from the alphoid centromere regions. They are not the actual regions involved, for instance, in causing Down's syndrome. We use repetitive, usually centromeric, probes.

Dr. Grzeschik: As well as these centromeric probes, people use a sort of collection of cloned DNA covering the length of the chromosome. Again I have to stress that with both techniques one does not cover the whole chromosome. One either has several islands on the chromosome or one piece near the centromere, so one is essentially looking for trisomy of fragments of chromosome 21.

Dr. Pollak: What percentage of cystic fibrosis (CF) mutation have you detected in your background population?

Dr. Grzeschik: The best figures from our country come from Schmidtke's group in this city. They have estimated the frequency of the Delta F mutation to be 77.3%.

Dr. Golbus: I believe that CF is going to represent a good example of what we call reversed genetics. The Delta 508 deletion has turned out not to be as promising as had been hoped. In the United States, we find a tremendous variability in the incidence of this mutation within different ethnic groups. The hope that there would only be a few more CF mutations has not proved true. We now know of about 30 mutations, none of which have a percentage that runs as high as 3%. This information will increase the ability to identify the protein that is made by the CF gene, and whereas we may not be able to do DNA screening of the population, when we have this protein and find out its real function, we may be able to have population screening based on the protein.

Dr. Grzeschik: We need to consider the consequences of such screening. Families with CF support CF research mainly to get improved treatment, not specifically to be able to have their pregnancies terminated. We should concentrate our efforts on treatment possibilities, rather than just identifying pregnancies to be terminated.

Dr. Golbus: The American Society of Genetics looked at this issue and came up with the statement that they did not believe that screening the population was appropriate at this time. The tendency to screen widely for the condition in the United States is largely the result of commercial pressure and clearly not the belief of the genetics community.

On another matter, the ability of the polymerase chain reaction to amplify DNA from single oocytes raises the problem of contamination. Even a single cell can lead to amplification of the wrong genome.

Dr. Grzeschik: The only way to solve this at present is to be extremely careful with sampling. One could also identify the origin of the material using polymorphism. Highly informative RFLP is very useful in identifying the source of the DNA. The same method is also helpful in indirect DNA diagnosis since if one of the family members who is tested does not belong biologically to this family, then of course your diagnosis is incorrect.

Dr. Holzgreve: With regard to the use of probes to detect the most frequent trisomies, I feel that although the approach is attractive from a screening point of view, we would certainly miss those occasional cases that we encounter in prenatal diagnosis where there is an unexpected translocation or other rearrangement. These may not be identified even by the panel of probes you use. Thus careful karyotyping might still provide the maximum amount of information.

Dr. Golbus: There is no question that some abnormalities found by full karyotyping would be missed by *in situ* hybridization. But there are at least two instances where you might want to consider using this procedure. First, there are developing countries that do not have tissue culture facilities, where the ability to find 90% of the abnormalities would certainly be an improvement over their present situation. Secondly, in the industrialized nations there is pressure from younger women who want prenatal diagnosis that at present cannot be provided. There is no question that the cost of hybridization will be substantially less than karyotyping.

I should like to raise three further points. Will the amount of money devoted to the genome project significantly reduce the amount available for research in other areas? And do people really want all this information? Are we as a society ready to handle the possibility of identifying genes for many more conditions than have been studied up to now?

Dr. Grzeschik: The amount of money devoted to the search for the CF gene might well have been enough to map the whole of chromosome 7, since many groups worked in parallel and much information was discarded. The idea behind the genome project is to coordinate the efforts and to make valuable mapping information available generally, not just to specific groups. As for the readiness of society to know about all disease genes, I see this from the patient's view. The diseases that have been investigated up to now are the most attractive from the medical and scientific point of view. The very rare diseases have not attracted so much attention, but cause great distress to small numbers of people. If one had a map as projected in the genome approach, even small groups that are interested in specific rare mutations would have a sound basis for tackling the problem.

Perinatology, edited by Erich Saling,
Nestlé Nutrition Workshop Series, Vol. 26,
Nestec, Ltd., Vevey/Raven Press, Ltd.,
New York © 1992.

Fetal Therapy

Mitchell S. Golbus

*Department of Obstetrics, Gynecology and Reproductive Sciences,
University of California, San Francisco, School of Medicine, San Francisco,
California 94143–0720, USA*

The ultimate goal for prenatal diagnosis is treatment of the affected fetus to correct the defect. For many disorders it is unlikely that effective corrective or preventative therapy will be developed in the foreseeable future. Furthermore, in at least some metabolic disorders, irreversible fetal damage may have occurred by the time the prenatal diagnosis is made. It is possible, however, to outline therapeutic alternatives for the management of a number of fetal disorders that can be recognized *in utero.*

Most correctable malformations that can be diagnosed *in utero* are best managed by appropriate medical or surgical therapy after delivery at term. The full-term infant is better able than the prematurely delivered infant to tolerate surgery and anesthesia. Prenatal diagnosis may be important because many anomalies are associated with an excess of amniotic fluid, which may initiate premature labor. Therapy for the excess amniotic fluid or premature labor may allow the fetus to remain *in utero* longer and be born at term. Additionally, the delivery can be planned so that the necessary neonatologists, anesthesiologists, and pediatric surgeons are available.

There is a subset of fetal anomalies that requires correction *ex utero* as soon as possible after the diagnosis is made. For these, the risk of prematurity must be weighed against the risk of continued gestation. The principle in each case is that continued gestation would have progressive ill effects on the fetus.

Another subset of fetal disorders may influence the mode of delivery and require that a cesarean section be performed. One indication for cesarean delivery is an anomaly such that the fetus could not fit through the maternal pelvis during vaginal delivery. Occasionally, an elective cesarean section may be indicated for a malformation requiring immediate surgical correction in a sterile environment. Occasionally, infants are delivered who are at risk for a severe immunodeficiency state that would cause them to be unable to withstand infections. Such infants have been delivered by elective cesarean section to protect their sterility.

IN UTERO INTERVENTION

There is a subset of fetal deficiency states that may be alleviated by *in utero* treatment. These are conditions in which something vital to fetal well-being is not

23

present in sufficient quantity, and supplementation of the missing element would constitute medical therapy. The simplest method of supplying the fetus is to give the missing element to the mother and allow it to be transported across the placenta to the fetus. Two fetuses have been diagnosed *in utero* as having vitamin-dependent enzyme deficiencies and have been treated before birth. The first had a vitamin-B_{12}-responsive enzyme disorder (methylmalonic acidemia) (1), and the second had a biotin-dependent disorder (multiple carboxylase deficiency) (2). Each was treated by giving the mother massive doses of the required vitamin. Both of these children are developing normally, albeit taking huge daily supplements of the necessary vitamin. Another example of medicating the fetus via the mother has been the successful treatment of fetal heart rhythm irregularities by giving the mother digitalis. The digitalis crosses the placenta to the fetus and has returned the fetal heart rate to a normal pattern.

The list of substances that will be given therapeutically to the fetus *in utero* is certain to grow. For example, it may be possible to treat intrauterine growth retardation, in which a normal fetus is not receiving sufficient nutrition, by instilling nutrients into the amniotic sac. Scientists are investigating enzyme therapy for enzyme deficient children. If such techniques can be developed, supplying the missing enzyme to the fetus *in utero* would represent only one further technical step, and might prevent an irreversible collection and storage of the enzyme substrate.

SURGICAL FETAL THERAPY

The complement of medical therapy is, of course, surgical therapy. Correcting an anatomic malformation will be more difficult than providing a missing substrate, hormone, or medication to the fetus. The prenatally diagnosable anatomic malformations that warrant consideration for surgical therapy are those that interfere with fetal organ development and, if alleviated, would allow normal fetal development to proceed. The first malformations that I shall consider are (a) hydronephrosis secondary to an obstruction, (b) diaphragmatic hernia, and (c) hydrocephalus.

URINARY TRACT OBSTRUCTION

Obstructive fetal urinary tract malformations are being recognized with increasing frequency because fluid-filled masses are particularly easy to detect by sonography. Retained fetal urine may cause a large distended bladder (megacystis), fluid-filled ureters (hydroureters), and fluid accumulation in the kidneys (hydronephrosis). The increased fluid and back pressure interfere with fetal kidney development and may cause sufficient kidney damage to be incompatible with postnatal life. The lack of fetal urine excretion secondarily causes a decrease in the volume of amniotic fluid. The decreased amniotic fluid is associated with underdevelopment of the lungs. The severity of the damage depends on the degree and duration of the urinary outflow obstruction.

It has been observed that failure to take action often leads to the delivery at term of an infant who has neither sufficient functioning kidney tissue or lung capacity to survive. Therefore, the philosophy has developed that it may be advisable to relieve the obstruction at the earliest possible time (3). The concept is that continued obstruction will result in a kidney with such impaired development that survival is impossible, whereas relief of the obstruction may allow sufficient development to support postnatal life and allow "catch-up" development during early childhood.

A thorough ultrasonographic evaluation is the key factor in the management of fetal urinary obstruction. Identification of fetal urinary tract dilatation is not uncommon, especially prior to 24 weeks of gestation. However, this dilatation does not, by itself, reflect an obstruction compromising renal function. It is important to separate these entities from each other. The amount of amniotic fluid is very important. If an adequate amount of amniotic fluid is evident on ultrasound, it signifies reasonable fetal renal function and usually assures adequate pulmonary development. Oligohydramnios, on the other hand, signifies fetal urinary tract obstruction. It is imperative that a thorough sonographic evaluation be performed to rule out any additional significant anomaly or disease. A fetal karyotype should be done, because chromosomal abnormalities have been associated with urinary tract abnormalities and obstruction (4).

FETAL RENAL ASSESSMENT

In utero decompression of fetal hydronephrosis or early delivery for *ex utero* decompression is only beneficial for fetuses whose kidneys have not already suffered irreversible damage. Appropriate counseling and management, therefore, require accurate assessment of renal function, to allow selection of pregnancies likely to benefit from therapeutic intervention.

Renal dysplasia, defined as abnormal parenchymal development secondary to anomalous differentiation of mesonephric tissue, implies irreversible renal damage (5). The functional capacity of an affected kidney depends upon the extent and severity of the dysplasia. Cortical cysts are often, but not necessarily, present. Extensive cortical dysplasia makes unlikely any beneficial effect of decompression of urinary tract obstruction.

SONOGRAPHIC EVALUATION OF RENAL DYSPLASIA

Dysplastic kidneys are associated with renal cortical cysts and increased echogenicity. In our experience (6), visible cortical cysts have a sensitivity of 44% and specificity of 100% in predicting renal dysplasia. Increased echogenicity has a sensitivity of 57% and specificity of 89%. The severity of hydronephrosis is least predictive, with a sensitivity of 35% and specificity of 78%. The demonstration of renal cortical cysts has the highest predictive value for dysplasia among fetuses with obstructive uropathy. Among 34 kidneys with dysplasia, all 15 with sonographically

TABLE 1. *Prognostic criteria for fetal bilateral urinary tract obstruction*

Predicted function	Sonographic appearance of kidneys	Initial amniotic fluid status	Fetal urine		
			Na (mEq/ml)	Cl (mEq/ml)	Osmolarity (mosm/l)
Poor	Echogenic/cystic	Moderate to severely decreased	>100	>90	>210
Good	Normal/echogenic	Normal to moderately decreased	<100	<90	<210

visible cortical cysts were also highly echogenic. Ten other kidneys were echogenic without demonstrable cysts, however, and an additional nine dysplastic kidneys had neither sonographically visible cysts nor increased echogenicity. Thus, visualization of a kidney without demonstrable cysts or increased echogenicity does not exclude dysplasia.

BIOCHEMICAL AND PHYSIOLOGICAL EVALUATION

Because sonography is not able to identify all dysplastic kidneys and therefore cannot distinguish accurately those fetuses with bilateral urinary tract obstruction that can benefit from decompression from those that cannot, biochemical studies have been considered. Fetal urine is produced by the 13th gestational week and is an ultrafiltrate of fetal serum made hypotonic by selective tubular absorption of Na and Cl (7). In our retrospective experience (8) fetuses with hypotonic urine were later found to have good renal function, whereas those with isotonic urine were found to have poor function. Based on these results, prognostic criteria for identifying the fetuses with good function or with poor function have been generated (Table 1).

The most difficult problem in the management of the fetus with urinary tract obstruction has been the selection of the fetus that might benefit from *in utero* treatment. Study of the natural history of untreated obstruction has shown that the fetus with unilateral obstruction and the fetus with mild bilateral obstruction and normal amniotic fluid volume do not require *in utero* therapy (9). Also, the fetus that presents with severe oligohydramnios and severe dysplastic kidney changes seen by sonography is unlikely to benefit from *in utero* therapy (5). Between these extremes there is a gray zone where potentially fatal renal and pulmonary damage may be averted by intervention. Assessment of the functional potential of the obstructed fetal urinary tract has proven difficult. Indirect methods, such as sonographic determination of bladder filling and emptying (10) or stimulation of urine production by furosemide (11) have proven unreliable. The development of the prognostic criteria given above that predict the potential for recovery has greatly simplified counseling of families and the selection of appropriate management.

MANAGEMENT OF FETAL URINARY TRACT OBSTRUCTION

Patients who are referred for evaluation undergo a thorough real-time ultrasound examination. If other life-threatening abnormalities are identified, we counsel the parents about these findings and their significance. Most couples, at this time, elect to proceed with pregnancy termination.

If ultrasonography reveals no evidence of additional anomalies, the amount of amniotic fluid becomes the deciding factor in our management scheme. There are instances of hydramnios and dilated urinary tract systems, most often associated with unilateral obstruction. If the amniotic fluid volume is normal, the nature of the obstruction becomes paramount. Uncomplicated unilateral obstruction with a normal amniotic fluid volume does not warrant interventive decompression (10).

For bilateral urinary tract obstruction with normal amniotic fluid volumes, we do not recommend invasive intervention. If the hydronephrosis is sufficiently severe we accelerate pulmonary maturity with betamethasone and proceed with delivery between 32 and 34 weeks gestation by the vaginal route, unless cesarean section is dictated by other obstetric indications. Of some concern are two neonates who died of pulmonary hypoplasia with associated urinary tract obstruction yet had "adequate" amniotic fluid volumes throughout pregnancy. We have also reported cases in which the obstruction actually resolved with expectant management, and term deliveries resulted with normal neonatal urinary and pulmonary function (9).

Therapy for urinary tract obstruction is reserved for cases that demonstrate isolated bilateral urinary tract obstruction with oligohydramnios. We start with needle aspiration of the fetal bladder to determine the osmolarity of the urine and its Na and Cl concentrations, thus separating dysplastic kidneys from the nondysplastic ones. Patients whose fetuses have severe oligohydramnios and severe renal dysplasia are offered the options of early termination of the pregnancy or nonintervention.

TABLE 2. *Primary diagnosis and outcome in 87 fetuses treated by vesico-amniotic shunting*

Primary diagnosis[a]	No. of cases	% of total	No. of survivors	% Survival by diagnosis
Posterior urethral valve syndrome	25	28.7%	17	68%
Karyotype abnormality[b]	7	8%	0	0%
Renal dysplasia by ultrasound[b]	6	6.9%	0	0%
Urethral atresia	6	6.9%	1	17%
"Prune belly" syndrome	5	5.7%	1	20%
Uretero-pelvic obstruction	2	2.3%	2	100%
Unknown etiology	36	41.3%	11	30.6%
Total	87	100%	32	40.2%

[a] Primary diagnosis as confirmed by either antenatal or neonatal assessment or autopsy.
[b] Elective pregnancy termination.
Data from the *International Registry*, 1986, by Dr. Frank Manning, Winnipeg, Canada (with permission).

TABLE 3. *Presentation, open surgery management, and*

Case no.	Maternal history	Ultrasound findings	Urine Na, Cl, Osm/ Chromosomes
1	18 y o, G-1, P-0 Oligohydramnios persisted 15 wk., Presented at 19 wk. C/S at 35 wk.	Bilateral fetal hydronephrosis. Megacystis, dilated bladder neck; renal parenchyma: increased echogenicity	Na 99 mEq/l Cl 84 mEq/l Osm 235 46,XY
2	31 y o, G-1, P-0 Oligohydramnios pt normal for 9 wk.	Bilateral fetal hydronephrosis. Megacystis, dilated bladder neck	Na 88 mEq/l Cl 83 mEq/l Osm 255
3	19 y o, G-1, P-0 Oligohydramnios AF normal for 11 wk. Presented at 22 wk.	Bilateral fetal hydronephrosis. Megacystis; renal parenchyma: normal	Na 79 mEq/l Cl 71 mEq/l Osm 160 46,XX
4	35 y o, G-1, P-0 Oligohydramnios AF normal for 14 wk. Presented at 18 wk.	Bilateral fetal hydronephrosis. Megacystis; renal parenchyma: normal	Na 100 mEq/l Cl 91 mEq/l Osm 221 46,XX
5	28 y o, G-4, P-3 Oligohydramnios AF normal for 10 wk. Presented at 22 wk. C/S at 32 wk.	Bilateral fetal hydronephrosis. Megacystis; thorax bell-shaped, renal parenchyma: increased echogenicity	Na 100 mEq/l Cl 92 mEq/l Osm 215 46,XY
6	25 y o, G-1, P-0 Oligohydramnios Presented at 23.5 wk. C/S at 25.5 wk.	Bilateral fetal hydronephrosis. Megacystis; kidneys: unilateral small cysts	Na 74 mEq/l Cl 71 mEq/l Osm 165 46,XX

The outcome of these pregnancies, in our experience, has been very poor with no survivors (9).

If the menstrual age is less than 32 weeks, amniotic fluid volume is decreased, and adequate renal function is present, then the UCSF team offers vesico-amniotic shunting. Each mother is sedated with intravenous diazepam prior to infiltration of her skin with lidocaine for placement of a needle and a catheter into the fetal bladder. Uterine activity is monitored and ritodrine hydrochloride given if significant uterine contractions occur. The placement of a permanent, double pigtailed fetal bladder catheter allows shunting of fetal urine into the amniotic cavity and prevents pulmonary hypoplasia (8). Data are sent to the Fetal Surgery Registry where 87 cases of fetal obstructive uropathy treated by *in utero* placement of a chronic vesico-amniotic shunt have been registered (12). Thirty-five out of the 87 treated fetuses survived (40.2%). In 13 cases (14.9%) pregnancy was electively terminated after shunt placement (Table 2). Seven of these 13 cases (8%) showed an abnormal karyotype subsequent to treatment. Of the remaining 74 pregnancies that were allowed to continue, 35 infants survived (47.3%).

As vesico-amniotic catheters are often displaced or blocked, requiring *in utero* replacement of the catheter, patients at UCSF of less than 28 menstrual weeks are offered open fetal surgery under general anesthesia. The uterus is opened in an area *outcome in six fetuses with bilateral hydronephrosis*

Procedure	Neonatal outcome	Long term
Bilateral ureterostomies at 20 wk.	Neonatal death. Pulmonary hypoplasia; Renal dysplasia	—
Fetal bladder marsupialization at 24 wk.	Live-born. Good pulmonary function	Alive. 3 years old; Renal insufficiency
Fetal bladder marsupialization at 23 wk.	Live-born. Good pulmonary function; Normal renal function	Died unrelated causes 9 months old.
Fetal bladder marsupialization at 18 wk.	Live-born. Good pulmonary function	Alive. 2 years old; Normal renal function
Fetal bladder marsupialization at 22 wk.	Neonatal death. Pulmonary hypoplasia; Renal dysplasia	—
Fetal bladder marsupialization at 24 wk. Abnormalities: hypoplastic lungs, renal dysplasia	Neonatal death at 25.5 wk with multiple congenital anomalies	—

AF, amniotic fluid; C/S, cesarean section.

chosen by sonographic evaluation, the lower abdominal wall of the fetus is exposed, and the fetal bladder is marsupialized. The UCSF experience with the first six such open human fetal procedures is summarized in Table 3.

One fetus underwent bilateral ureterostomies and the other five had bladder marsupializations. Five pregnancies proceeded to cesarean delivery at 32 to 35 menstrual weeks. Neither intraoperative complications nor long-term maternal morbidity occurred. Three of these pregnancies had normal amniotic fluid volumes after intervention and had normal pulmonary function at birth. The outcome varied in the three surviving children: one died of unrelated reasons at 9 months of age with normal renal function, one has normal renal function at 22 months, and the third started manifesting renal failure at 2 years of age and required renal transplantation at 4 years.

The three neonatal deaths were all due to pulmonary hypoplasia and renal dysplasia. On sonography, all three had increased renal parenchymal echogenicity. One pregnancy never had a normal amniotic fluid volume after decompression and a second showed a deformed tiny chest cavity due to the long period of oligohydramnios before decompression. Pregnancy number 6 was terminated at 26 weeks when recurrence of oligohydramnios and a dilated bladder made a second intervention necessary. When fetal exploration showed anal atresia and a cloacal abnormality in this female fetus, the mother wished to terminate the pregnancy. Autopsy findings included lung immaturity, renal dysplasia, and multiple abnormalities.

Our current selection criteria, including favorable fetal urine electrolytes and osmolarity, sonographically normal renal parenchyma and oligohydramnios, would have excluded from treatment the three fetuses who died as neonates and the fetus who later developed renal failure.

DIAPHRAGMATIC HERNIA

Congenital diaphragmatic hernia is usually an isolated anomaly in an otherwise normal full-term infant. The abnormality is a failure of the diaphragm to form and to separate the abdominal wall and chest cavities. The bowel and other abdominal contents herniate into the chest. Surgical correction consists of placing the herniated bowel back in the abdomen and closing the defect in the diaphragm. However, approximately 80% of these infants die of lung underdevelopment caused by lung compression during the last half of gestation (13). The incidence of congenital diaphragmatic hernia is between 1:2,500 and 1:5,000 newborns, so that 700 to 1,400 affected children are born annually in the United States. Despite marked advances in neonatal anesthetic, surgical, and respiratory care over the last two decades, the mortality rate of this anomaly has not changed.

A study of Adzick *et al.* (14) surveyed collaborative results of 94 fetuses diagnosed with congenital diaphragmatic hernias. Prenatal diagnosis was made in 88 of the cases and retrospectively appreciated in six cases. In 66% of these cases, the mother was referred for an ultrasound examination for uterine size larger than dates, and polyhydramnios was noted in conjunction with congenital diaphragmatic hernia. Approximately 20% were diagnosed at the time of a routine obstetric ultrasound evaluation. In 97% of the cases, the diagnosis could be made with ultrasound alone or in conjunction with an amniogram or single section computerized tomography scan (14 cases). Polyhydramnios was present in 76% of the cases.

The survival results in these infants were discouraging. Ninety percent of the cases had optimal perinatal care, including maternal transport, planned delivery, immediate resuscitation, pediatric surgical consultation, etc. However, only 20% of these infants survived, and three of these developed severe bronchopulmonary dysplasia requiring prolonged postoperative respiratory support. The need for a thorough prenatal evaluation was evidenced by a 16% rate of lethal associated anomalies, mostly cardiac, chromosomal, or CNS. The presence of late gestation polyhydramnios was found to be a prognostic indicator. The survival rate for infants with polyhydramnios was 11% and for those without polyhydramnios, a more encouraging 55%.

To date, *in utero* correction of a diaphragmatic hernia has been attempted on a few fetuses referred to the University of California, San Francisco, Fetal Treatment Program. Upon referral, extensive counseling was performed and most couples have not requested a surgical attempt at closure. The first two that have been attempted were evaluated and neither of these fetuses were found to have coexisting anomalies, and both had normal karyotypes. At the time of surgery, both fetuses were found to have the entire liver in the chest cavity, and attempts to replace the liver into the abdomen proved fatal. These were felt to have been inoperable, postnatally. Additional experience is still at an early stage but has now produced the first surviving neonates.

FETAL VENTRICULOMEGALY

Hydrocephalus of prenatal origin occurs in 0.2% of all deliveries. It represents a failure of normal cerebrospinal fluid dynamics so that this fluid accumulates in the ventricles, causing them to enlarge and cause pressure atrophy of the brain (15). The diagnosis of ventriculomegaly has been made by ultrasound as early as the 13th menstrual week (16). The choroid plexus fills the ventricles until 20 weeks so that excess fluid is usually apparent. After 20 weeks, the most frequently used measure of ventriculomegaly is the LVW/HW ratio, which is the ratio of the displacement of the lateral wall of the ventricle (LVW) to the hemispheric width (HW). Filly and Callen have suggested a more sensitive measure: that of the displacement of the medial wall of the lateral ventricle toward the midline (17).

Trials using ventriculo-amniotic (V-A) shunts in human pregnancies by Clewell *et al.* (18) or multiple aspiration by Frigoletto *et al.* (19) were fraught with complications such as blockage and infection. A review in 1986 by Manning *et al.* (12) showed that 34 out of 39 fetuses shunted for hydrocephalus survived, but 22 of these had varying degrees of deficit.

Because there is no clear benefit to intrauterine shunting for hydrocephalus at the present time, operative candidates must be carefully selected. Detailed ultrasonography should be performed to look for associated anomalies. Karyotyping should be performed and amniotic fluid alpha-fetoprotein should be assessed to aid in the diagnosis of neural tube defects. A careful history should be taken from the mother and testing performed to rule out infections such as congenital rubella, toxoplasmosis, cytomegalovinus, and syphilis. Because progression of ventricular enlargement is unusual, stable ventriculomegaly should be followed to term. Progressive lesions in extremely premature fetuses might be considered for intrauterine treatment. However, experience thus far seems to indicate that although V-A shunting may improve survival, especially in cases of aqueductal stenosis, the shunts are subject to frequent mishaps without clear benefit to cerebral function. Until there are better diagnostic criteria for selecting the at-risk fetus who could be helped by shunting, there is a self-imposed moratorium on ventricular shunting.

COMMENTARY

The potential for *in utero* correction of some birth defects gives added significance to the rapidly expanding field of prenatal diagnosis. Therapeutic decisions will require a thorough evaluation of the fetus beyond accurate anatomic definition of any malformation being considered for therapy. Because it is known that malformations often occur as part of a syndrome, a search for associated abnormalities is necessary to avoid delivering a neonate with one corrected anomaly, but other unrecognized disabling or lethal abnormalities.

A major issue has been whether it would be possible to open the uterus and operate upon the fetus without jeopardizing the mother and/or fetus. The threat of precipitating preterm labor and abortion remain the principal barriers to such fetal surgery. Limited experience with surgical exposure of the human fetus for even a minor procedure in the 1960s was so unfavorable that the procedure was abandoned. Over the last few years extensive research on fetal surgery in models, particularly monkeys, has resulted in improved techniques of anesthesia, surgery, and labor inhibition. These advances have now been employed in performing the first successful *in utero* fetal surgical procedures, and a milestone has been passed.

The benefits and risks of fetal diagnosis and therapy will have to be carefully evaluated and weighed, keeping in mind that two patients are being treated. Assessment for the fetus will be relatively straightforward: the risk of the procedure and/or medication versus the benefit of correction or amelioration of the deleterious condition. This last factor will depend on the severity of the condition and its predictable consequences on survival and quality of life. Assessment for the mother will be more difficult. Her health usually will not be affected by the fetal disorder, but she will have to bear some risk from the therapy attempt.

Our ability to diagnose fetal birth defects has achieved considerable sophistication. Treatment of several fetal conditions has now proven to be feasible, and treatment of more complicated defects will expand as techniques for fetal intervention improve. The concept that the fetus is a patient, an individual whose disorders are a proper subject for medical therapy, has been established.

REFERENCES

1. Ampola MG, Mahoney MJ, Nakamura E, Tanaka K. Prenatal therapy of a patient with vitamin-B_{12}-responsive methylamalonic acidemia. *N Engl J Med* 1975;293:313–7.
2. Packman S, Cowan MJ, Golbus MS, *et al*. Prenatal treatment of biotin responsive multiple carboxylase deficiency. *Lancet* 1982;1:1435–9.
3. Harrison MR, Filly RA, Parer JT, *et al*. Management of the fetus with a urinary tract malformation. *JAMA* 1981;246:635–9.
4. Frydman M, Magenis RE, Mohandas TK, *et al*. Chromosome abnormalities in infants with prune belly anomaly: association with trisomy 18. *Am J Med Genet* 1983;15:145–8.
5. Bernstein J. The morphogenesis of renal parenchymal maldevelopment (renal dysplasia). *Pediatr Clin North Am* 1971;18:395–407.
6. Mahoney BS, Filly RA, Callen PW, *et al*. Sonographic evaluation of renal dysplasia. *Radiology* 1984;152:143–6.
7. McGrory WW. *Development of renal function in utero*, Ch 2. Cambridge, MA: Harvard Univ Press, 1972;51–78.
8. Golbus MS, Filly RA, Callen PW, *et al*. Fetal urinary tract obstruction: management and selection for treatment. *Semin Perinatol* 1985;9:91–7.
9. Harrison MR, Golbus MS, Filly RA, *et al*. Management of the fetus with congenital hydronephrosis. *J Pediatr Surg* 1982;17:728–42.

10. Campbell S, Wladimiroff JW, Dewhurst CJ. The antenatal measurement of fetal urine production. *J Obstet Gynecol Br Cwlth* 1973;80:680–6.
11. Wladimiroff JW. Effect of furosemide on fetal urine production. *Br J Obstet Gynaecol* 1975;82: 221–4.
12. Manning FA, Harrison MR, Rodeck C, Members of the International Fetal Medicine and Surgery Society. Catheter shunts for fetal hydronephrosis and hydrocephalus: report of the International Fetal Surgery Registry. *N Engl J Med* 1986;315:336–40.
13. Harrison MR, Bjordal RI, Langmark F, Knutrud O. Congenital diaphragmatic hernia: the hidden mortality. *J Pediatr Surg* 1978;13:227–30.
14. Adzick NS, Harrison MR, Blick PL, *et al.* Diaphragmatic hernia in the fetus: prenatal diagnosis and outcome in 94 cases. *J Pediatr Surg* 1985;20:357–61.
15. Epstein M Hydrocephalus. In: Ravitch MM, Welch KJ, Benson CD, *et al.*, eds. *Pediatric Surgery*, 3rd ed. Chicago: Year Book Medical Publishers, Inc., 1979.
16. Hudgins RJ, Edwards MSB, Goldstein R, *et al.* Natural history of fetal ventriculomegaly. *Pediatrics* 1988;82:692–7.
17. Fiske CE, Filly RA, Callen PW. Sonographic measurement of lateral ventricular width in early ventricular dilation. *J Clin Ultrasound* 1981;9:303–7.
18. Clewell WH, Johnson ML, Meier PR, *et al.* A surgical approach to the treatment of fetal hydrocephalus. *N Engl J Med* 1982;306:1320–5.
19. Frigoletto FD, Birnholz JC, Greene MF. Antenatal treatment of hydrocephalus by ventriculoamniotic shunting. *N Engl J Med* 1982;306:2496–7.

DISCUSSION

Dr. Pollak: I was very interested in the results of your diaphragmatic hernia babies. You pointed out that one of the major problems is hypoplasia of the lung. What happened to your patients' lungs after surgery?

Dr. Golbus: Diaphragmatic hernia occurs very early in development at a time when the number of bronchial branches is determined. Even if the intrathoracic mass is removed, it is too late for any growth of new bronchial branches. However, the lung is capable of developing more villi off each of the existing branches, and in as little as 5 to 6 weeks there is enough catch-up in lung growth for the fetus to be able to breathe.

Dr. Marini: Would you comment about amniotic pressure and lung hypoplasia. We usually assume that there is high amniotic fluid pressure in these cases, but recently Nicolini in England (1) showed that there is low pressure in some of these cases. Could we treat very early during pregnancy by giving infusions into the amniotic cavity?

Dr. Golbus: I do not think amniotic infusions would be likely to help in cases where there is a mass in the chest, but certainly in cases of oligohydramnios of unknown etiology we will end up with hypoplastic lungs if we do nothing. We have tried infusions and have had some successes and some failures. On balance we feel such treatment is worth trying in oligohydramnios of unknown etiology.

Dr. Gold: One of the biggest problems in open fetal surgery is that it requires a corporeal cesarean section. This is a big decision for the mother to take. Can you comment on this? I have heard and read that results with congenital diaphragmatic hernia are disappointing, so the question of the operation on the uterus needs careful examination.

Dr. Golbus: With regard to the operation, we tell the patients that since they are going to have a classical incision they will need to have a cesarean in every future pregnancy. We counsel very strongly that we are not just talking about one operation but three or four or as many as there will be children. I agree that open surgery involves a whole new consideration because risk to the mother is involved, not just to the fetus. The majority of patients we counsel decide not to proceed. With regard to prognosis, we have performed eight *in utero* diaphragmatic hernia repairs. The first four died, and of the second four, three were delivered alive but one subsequently died of an unrelated cause.

Dr. Guesry: What is the optimal time for surgery?

Dr. Golbus: The optimal time is different for different conditions. For bladder obstruction, operation can take place as early as 18 weeks, since the procedure is very brief and well tolerated. Diaphragmatic hernia surgery cannot be done until about 24 weeks since before that time the fetus cannot tolerate the procedure, which lasts for an hour at least even with practice.

Dr. Van Geijn: How would you compare intrauterine surgery at 24 to 25 weeks with early delivery and neonatal surgery, with life support by ECMO or ventilation?

Dr. Golbus: I am not an expert on ECMO but the Boston group looked at their diaphragmatic hernia neonates with and without ECMO and did not find it very helpful. We have ECMO and we use it, but I don't think we know yet how helpful it is going to be. With regard to other prenatally diagnosed conditions *in utero* transplantation may offer some hope of success. We and others have been able to do successful *in utero* transplants in a mouse model and our group has also published results of successful rhesus monkey allogenic transplantation. In the successful rhesus model there was a range of 5–10% of donor cells in the recipient's peripheral circulation after birth, in all cell lines. Although this may be sufficient to correct an enzymopathy, it is not sufficient to correct a hemoglobinopathy. However, clinically we are going to be transplanting in a situation in which there is a disease, and this may give the donor cells a competitive advantage and increase their engraftment. We need to be transplanting at the time when the fetus is seeding the marrow, about 20 weeks. If we seed our donor cells later than this it will probably be too late both for immunologic (rejection) and hematopoietic reasons.

REFERENCE

1. Nicolini U, Fisk NM, Rodeck CH, Talbert DG, Wigglesworth JS. Low amniotic pressure in oligohydramnios. Is this the cause of pulmonary hypoplasia? *Am J Obstet Gynecol* 1989;161:1098–101.

Perinatology, edited by Erich Saling,
Nestlé Nutrition Workshop Series, Vol. 26,
Nestec, Ltd., Vevey/Raven Press, Ltd.,
New York © 1992.

Embryonic and Fetal Circulation Studied by Transvaginal Color Doppler

Asim Kurjak and Ivica Zalud

*Ultrasonic Institute, University of Zagreb, "Dr. Josip Kajfes" Hospital,
Pavleka Miskine 64, WHO Collaborating Centre for Diagnostic Ultrasound,
41000 Zagreb, Yugoslavia*

Ultrasound is already an essential component of obstetric evaluation, but is gaining even more attention as Doppler techniques open new avenues into the diagnosis of blood flow disturbances in the fetus. Some investigators claim that Doppler is the biggest advance in fetal medicine in years (1). The role of fetal and uteroplacental blood flow studies is now well established in obstetric management, but until now there has been no reliable way to measure blood flow in the embryonic period non-invasively. Transvaginal color Doppler is a recently developed diagnostic tool that allows us to look closely at early embryonic development and to make blood flow studies in embryonic and fetal vessels.

PATIENTS AND METHODS

The study included 114 pregnant women volunteers whose gestational age ranged between 5 and 14 weeks. They were recruited from patients scheduled for termination of pregnancy on request. An additional 31 patients with pathologic early pregnancies were examined. Seventeen of these had an ultrasonically diagnosed blighted ovum, 11 had missed abortion, and in three cases a molar pregnancy was diagnosed.

All patients were examined with a 5 MHz transvaginal probe and the equipment employed was an Aloka Color Doppler, models SSD-350 and SSD-680 (Aloka Co., Japan). A condom and gel were placed over the head of the transducer, and the probe was then introduced gently into the vagina with the patient placed in the lithotomy position. After visualization of the pelvic anatomy by B-mode sonography, superimposed color Doppler was used to detect blood flow. The red or blue color indicated the vascular region to be examined by the pulsed Doppler technique for flow velocity waveform analysis. Peak systolic and end-diastolic Doppler shifts were recorded and the Pourcelot resistance index (RI) was calculated (2). This angle-independent index is believed to be a good assessor of downstream vascular

TABLE 1. *Resistance index of the uterine artery in the first trimester of pregnancy (n = 145)*

Patients	*n*	mean RI	2 SD
Normal pregnancy	114	0.81	0.11
Blighted ovum	17	0.77	0.13
Missed abortion	11	0.69	0.09
Mola hydatidosa	3	0.76	0.07

RI, Pourcelot resistance index.

resistance. On each record five separate cardiac cycles were examined and the mean value was calculated. The mean duration of the procedure was 10 min. The spatial-peak temporal average intensity was about 80 mW/cm^2, which is well within the highest limit recommended by the United States Food and Drug Administration for use in fetal medicine.

In all patients we tried to obtain signals from both the uterine arteries and the intervillous space. In 114 patients with normal pregnancies, additional analysis of signals from the umbilical artery and fetal aorta were performed. Fetal brain circulation was also investigated.

RESULTS

Uterine Arteries

Color Doppler signal from both uterine arteries could easily be seen in all patients just lateral to the cervix at the level of the cervicocorporeal junction of the uterus. The calculated resistance indices for the two groups of patients (normal and pathologic intrauterine pregnancy) are given in (Table 1). RI values ranged from 0.64 to 0.95, but statistical comparison of mean RI values for the various subgroups studied (normal pregnancy—mean RI 0.81 ± 0.11; blighted ovum—mean RI 0.77 ± 0.13; missed abortion—mean RI 0.69 ± 0.09; molar pregnancy—mean RI 0.76 ± 0.07) did not reveal any significant difference between the values obtained.

Intervillous Space

A color signal seen within a hyperechoic area in close proximity to the gestational sac was considered to be due to intervillous blood flow. When a consistent color signal was obtained in that region, a clear flow velocity waveform of high velocity and low resistance was always easily obtained (Fig. 1). Color flow signals were visualized in 40% of cases at 5 weeks gestation and in 100% of cases from the 7th

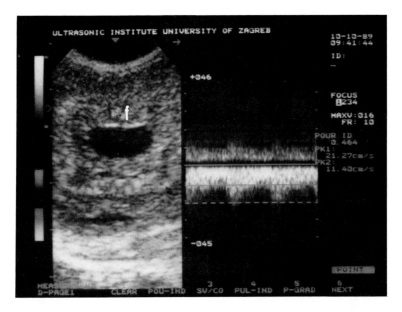

FIG. 1. Intervillous blood flow detected by transvaginal color Doppler at 5 weeks of gestation. Waveform analysis showed increased diastolic flow and low resistance (*right*). f, intervillous color flow.

week of gestation onward (Table 2). Mean RI values were 0.37 ± 0.08 in normal pregnancies, 0.34 ± 0.05 in blighted ovum pregnancies, 0.41 ± 0.07 in the cases of missed abortion, and 0.39 ± 0.11 in molar pregnancies. It should be stressed that in seven cases of missed abortion and five cases of blighted ovum we were unable to detect any intervillous flow.

TABLE 2. *Visualization rate by color Doppler signal of uterine artery, intervillous space, umbilical artery, fetal aorta, and intracranial circulation (n = 114)*

Weeks	n	A. uterina	Intervillous space	A. umbilicalis	Aorta	Brain
5	10	100%	4 (40%)	0	0	0
6	17	100%	9 (53%)	5 (29%)	0	0
7	25	100%	100%	100%	6 (24%)	0
8	14	100%	100%	100%	13 (93%)	0
9	5	100%	100%	100%	100%	0
10	7	100%	100%	100%	100%	0
11	3	100%	100%	100%	100%	0
12	17	100%	100%	100%	100%	7 (41%)
13	12	100%	100%	100%	100%	10 (83%)
14	4	100%	100%	100%	100%	4 (100%)

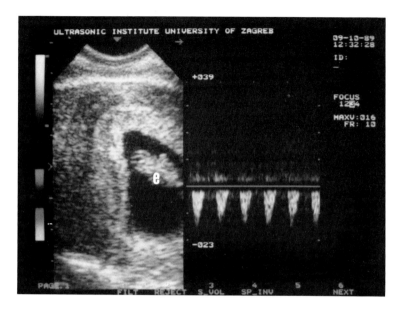

FIG. 2. Aortic blood flow detected at 8 weeks of gestation. Waveform analysis showed prominent systolic flow and no diastolic flow (*right*). e, embryo.

Umbilical Artery

Doppler color signals from the umbilical artery can only occasionally be seen at the 6th gestational week (29%), but are consistently obtained from the 7th gestational week onward (Table 2). During the period under investigation neither diastolic flow in umbilical arteries nor signals from the umbilical vein could be identified. This finding can be explained on the basis of slow, low volume umbilical cord flow at that gestational age which is below detectability with the present color Doppler sensitivity and 100 Hz high-pass filter pulse-wave Doppler.

Fetal Aorta

The fetal aorta can be visualized using transvaginal color Doppler from the 7th week of gestation in 24% of cases, and from 9 weeks onward in 100% of cases (Table 2). Waveform analysis showed no diastolic flow and a high regular systolic Doppler shift (Fig. 2).

Intracranial Circulation

It was possible to obtain clear and persistent intracranial color flow signals from 12 weeks of gestation onward. Small velocity flow with a notable diastolic component was seen (Table 2).

DISCUSSION

Two-dimensional ultrasonography allows direct assessment of the biometric, morphologic, and dynamic status of the fetus. The use of the recently developed Doppler techniques allows access to another type of information, the measurement of circulatory flows in the fetal as well as the maternal blood vessels. Although investigators have focused mainly on late second and third trimester pregnancy, Doppler studies have recently expanded to the first trimester as well (3–11). Its overall value in early pregnancy has yet to be established. It has been found that Doppler waveform patterns in the first trimester differ markedly from those found later in pregnancy (6). For example, the umbilical artery waveform has no diastolic component early in the first trimester under physiological conditions. This contrasts with the third trimester, when absent diastolic flow is associated with poor fetal outcome (7). Diastolic flow begins to increase around the 12th to 17th week, indicating the decrease in placental resistance.

Three kinds of Doppler equipment are presently used in obstetrics: continuous-wave Doppler (CWD), pulsed-wave Doppler (PWD), and color Doppler-coded imaging (CD). The CWD can use a simple and relatively cheap hand probe or it can be coupled with an imaging sonographic transducer or built into sonographic equipment. The PWD is commonly built into imaging sonographic equipment, where the Doppler beam is coaxial or at a variable angle with the sonographic image. The CD has until now been of limited use due to the cost of the equipment. However, it seems that color Doppler could increase the reproducibility of measurements, especially in the maternal circulation. With this modality it is possible to visualize even small vessels clearly, thus enabling accurate placing of pulsed Doppler sample volume. Furthermore, the visualization of flow direction yields information on flow profile. Color Doppler could reaffirm the value of volume flow measurement. Since there is no difference between the vessel diameter measured on B-mode and flow width, the vessel diameter can be accurately measured even in situations when the investigated vessel lies parallel to the ultrasound beam. Such cases are optimal for flow measurement. With good quality of Doppler signal and accurate diameter measurement the accuracy of volume flow measurement could be significantly improved (3).

We have combined color and pulsed-wave Doppler transvaginal sonography. The combination has given us the possibility of screening the vascularization of the entire pelvis rapidly. Only in cases when a color signal is detected away from major pelvic vessels has the time-consuming off-line pulse wave Doppler measurement been undertaken. The trophoblast invades the maternal tissues, and it is possible to get very high blood flow from the maternal arteries into the spaces around them. It is thus worth using this vascular signature of intervillous blood flow as a way confirming early pregnancy development. In this study the signals from the intervillous space umbilical artery and uterine arteries were easily obtained, but we were unable to detect any statistically significant difference in blood flow between normal and pathologic intrauterine pregnancies. This finding does not corroborate observations of

Schaaps and Soyeur (6), whose scanning technique was obviously different (they were unable to detect flow in the normal trophoblast). Thus much more standardized, probably multicenter, work is required before final conclusions can be drawn.

To sum up, embryonic and fetal vessels can easily be visualized by transvaginal color Doppler, and the pulsed Doppler beam can thus easily be directed at the vessel of interest. Color Doppler has been found to be particularly useful in demonstrating intervillous blood flow, flow in the fetal aorta and the intracranial circulation, as well as the uterine artery blood flow. If pulsed Doppler alone is used, the localization of blood flow is a time-consuming and relatively difficult procedure. The guidance of a pulsed Doppler beam by transvaginal color Doppler helps to locate areas of the most abundant flow and makes examination much faster and more accurate.

REFERENCES

1. D'Agincourt L. Doppler opens new paths into fetal evaluation. *Diagn Imaging* 1988;10:110.
2. Pourcelot L. Applications cliniques de l'examen Doppler transcutane. In: Peronneau P, ed. *Velocimetrie ultrasonore Doppler*. Paris: Seminaire INSERM, 1975;213.
3. Kurjak A, Alfirevic Z, Miljan M. Conventional and color Doppler in the assessment of fetal and maternal circulation. *Ultrasound Med Biol* 1988;14:337.
4. Kurjak A, Miljan M, Jurkovic D, Alfirevic Z, Zalud I. Color Doppler in the assessment of fetomaternal circulation. *Rech Gynecol* 1989;1:269.
5. Kurjak A, Jurkovic D, Alfirevic Z, Zalud I. Transvaginal color Doppler imaging. *J Clin Ultrasound* 1990;18:227.
6. Schaaps JP, Soyeur D. Pulsed Doppler on a vaginal probe. Necessity, convenience, or luxury? *J Ultrasound Med* 1989;8:315.
7. Hata K, Hata T, Senoh D, Aoki S, Takamiya O, Kitao M. Umbilical artery blood flow velocity waveforms and associations with fetal abnormality. *Gynecol Obstet Invest* 1989;27:179.
8. Schulman H. The clinical implication of Doppler ultrasound analysis of the uterine and umbilical arteries. *Am J Obstet Gynecol* 1987;156:889.
9. Trudinger BJ, Giles WB, Cook M, *et al.* Fetal umbilical artery flow velocity waveforms and placental resistance: clinical significance. *Br J Obstet Gynaecol* 1985;92:23.
10. Campbell S, Diaz-Recasens J, Griffin DR, *et al.* New Doppler technique for assessing uteroplacental blood flow. *Lancet* 1983;1:675.
11. Kurjak A, ed. *Measurements of fetal blood flow*. Rome: CIC, 1984.

DISCUSSION

Dr. Pollak: Could you expand your remarks on the reduced cerebral blood flow in growth retardation?

Dr. Kurjak: This was outside the scope of my presentation. However, we are studying various vessels with conventional color Doppler in our high-risk patients, including the uterine artery, the umbilical artery, the descending part of the fetal aorta, and the fetal cerebral arteries, to see if we can identify a brain-sparing effect. If there is abnormal blood flow in the fetomaternal vessels, the vessels of immediate interest are the cerebral or carotid arteries. The earliest sign of a dangerous situation in the fetus, whatever maternal complication is present, is reduced or absent diastolic flow, and there is an obvious difference between normal diastolic flow in the middle cerebral artery in normally oxygenated fetuses and reduced blood flow in growth-retarded fetuses.

Dr. Dawes: Does color Doppler improve the quantitative measurement of blood flow? And does it make the measurement quicker?

Dr. Kurjak: It certainly improves quantitative measurement but there are still many sources of error in trying to calculate volume of blood flow per kg fetal weight. However I believe that color Doppler will make such measurements more accurate and reproducible. The measurements can also be made much more quickly since the color can guide us to the structure of interest, after which we can superimpose pulsed Doppler for a brief period to get the required information.

Dr. Dawes: I noticed that on one or two occasions you had flows in opposite directions, presumably concurrent artery and vein.

Dr. Kurjak: Iliac arteries produce various blood flow patterns as part of their normal Doppler signature. This is a well-known phenomenon and I believe it results from the high peripheral resistance in the leg vessels producing a reversed signal in the pelvic vessels.

Dr. Hope: I am worried that abnormal middle cerebral artery waveforms could be caused by incomplete insonation of the vessel, and that management decisions are being made on the basis of these measurements.

Dr. Kurjak: Color Doppler always produces very typical signals and gives excellent orientation for the sample volume. So we visualize the vessel first and then put the sample volume inside the vessel. I am not worried that we are mistakenly identifying abnormal waveforms.

Dr. Hope: But I find the reproducibility of pulsed Doppler examinations of the neonatal head after birth worryingly poor.

Dr. Kurjak: Pulsed Doppler is completely different.

Dr. Hope: One can see the middle cerebral artery quite clearly in black and white and put the appropriate cursor in the appropriate place. What I am worried about is making management decisions based on reduced diastolic flow in the fetal brain. I don't think anyone has shown that intervention is necessary, or indeed has tested whether it is a reproducible finding. I don't know any data that confirm your assumptions that this finding means that the fetus should be delivered. You are presumably going to deliver many preterm babies on the basis of a finding that is incompletely understood at present.

Dr. Kurjak: I didn't say so. No single variable can be used to make the final decision. But if you have a growth-retarded fetus, already diagnosed by biometric measurements, if you have reduced pO_2 in fetal blood obtained from cordocentesis, and if you have noninvasive measurements of four fetal vessels all of which show abnormal size, then I don't think many of our colleagues would wait and see. There are several papers, (1,2), particularly from the Rotterdam center, showing that cerebral blood flow is a better index of fetal status than the others currently available.

Dr. Hope: I fully accept that it is a sign of fetal compromise. What I dispute is that the evidence exists for it to be used as a criterion for the *timing* of delivery, which is a different issue.

Dr. Dawes: What is the physiological basis for the changes you observe in the middle cerebral artery? Why do you think a reduction in diastolic flow occurs?

Dr. Kurjak: I believe that increased peripheral resistance is at least partly responsible.

Dr. Dawes: If you observe reduced flow in conjunction with hypoxemia and hypercapnia (which should cause cerebral vasodilatation) then there must be a reduction of arterial pressure. Is that a possible explanation? Or does anyone else have an explanation for this phenomenon? One of the difficulties in assessing intrauterine life is that you cannot measure pressure.

Dr. Kurjak: Your suggestion seems logical but we don't know the answer. We are only capable of recognizing a reduced or absent diastolic flow, or even a reversed flow, which from clinical experience most of us find very dangerous.

Dr. Rosén: In our studies on sheep, carotid flow has always been maintained even with the most severe degrees of asphyxia. My suggestion is that the lack of diastolic flow in the middle cerebral artery may be a sign of a decrease in myocardial performance with lowered blood pressure, which would interefere with the circulation in a peripheral artery but would not be detectable in a central artery.

Dr. Jouppila: I should like to stress that up to now we have no clinical marker in Doppler studies that indicates with near 100% certainty that the time for active management has arrived. Some fetuses can tolerate very high peripheral vascular resistance in the umbilical artery and descending aorta, and large decreases in end-diastolic flow in the middle cerebral artery, but tolerance may vary from only a few days to 2 to 3 weeks. The only marker I have seen that is invariably ominous is retrograde flow in the descending aorta or umbilical artery. We have seen this in about 12 cases and most of them died during the few days following the observation.

Dr. Saling: In our evaluation of severely growth-retarded fetuses studied by black and white Doppler, we found that in the group of cases in which there was zero flow we had higher mortality if we waited until the cardiotocograph became abnormal. I think a step-by-step diagnostic program should be used. The first step is the diagnosis of growth retardation; the second is a change in the ratio between the carotid artery and the aorta; the third is the appearance of zero flow in the fetal vessels. When this happens we have a very dangerous situation with high mortality. From our own experience the demonstration of abnormal Doppler patterns detects severe danger better than cardiotocography alone, though perhaps computed cardiotocography will improve on what we have at present.

Dr. Saling: Is the energy emitted during color Doppler comparable with black and white Doppler or greater? How dangerous is it?

Dr. Kurjak: Color Doppler is no more risky than conventional Doppler. For example the machine I use produces 80 mW/cm^2, which is well within the Food and Drug Administration limits. With pulsed Doppler, the ultrasonic beam is focused and energy is concentrated on the region of interest, but identifying this region is often time-consuming. When color is used, all vessels can be visualized simultaneously and thus the region of interest can be identified promptly and the energy dose reduced.

REFERENCES

1. Wladimiroff JW, Tonge HM, Stewart PA. Doppler ultrasound measurement of cerebral blood flow in the human fetus. *Br J Obstet Gynaecol* 1986;93:471.
2. Jouppila P, Kirkinen P. Increased vascular resistance in the descending aorta of the human fetus in hypoxia. *Br J Obstet Gynaecol* 1984;91:863

Perinatology, edited by Erich Saling,
Nestlé Nutrition Workshop Series, Vol. 26,
Nestec, Ltd., Vevey/Raven Press, Ltd.,
New York © 1992.

Antepartum Real-Time Magnetic Resonance Imaging in Obstetrics

Ian R. Johnson

*Department of Obstetrics and Gynaecology, City Hospital, Hucknall Road,
Nottingham NG5 1PB, England*

During the last 10 years magnetic resonance imaging (MRI) has gradually become established as a useful diagnostic procedure in clinical medicine. In the study of disease in the central nervous system, in the skeleton, and in many other organs in the body, high-resolution pictures have been obtained which are of inestimable use to those concerned with clinical management. Current imaging times still range from a few seconds to many minutes and although this is of no importance in the study of some structures within the body, in other areas it has caused significant problems. Fetal movement *in utero* during pregnancy lessens as the pregnancy progresses. Despite this, even near term there is enough movement to cause motional artifact on any imaging modality that takes more than milliseconds to acquire a picture. Conventional MRI has proved to be a disappointment because of this motional artifact. Echo planar imaging (EPI), a variant of MRI developed by Professor Peter Mansfield in Nottingham, acquires an image so quickly that it is suitable for use in obstetrics. Collaboration between the Departments of Physics and Obstetrics in Nottingham has resulted in the use of EPI to obtain pictures of fetuses at all stages of pregnancy.

METHODS

The concept of solving motional problems in MRI was first discussed by Mansfield in 1977 and 1978 (1,2). He proposed instantaneous data acquisition which he termed "snapshot." This process is now known as echo planar imaging. EPI has been used to image patients since 1983. The first obstetric patients were imaged early in 1988.

The images shown in this chapter were obtained using a prototype MRI system operating with a static magnetic field strength of 0.52 tesla. The Modulus Blipped Echo Planar Single Pulse Technique (MBEST), a variant of EPI, was used. This technique has been described elsewhere (3).

The patient lies supine on a moving bed that is pushed into the magnet. Because of the noise produced when the gradients switch the patient wears headphones for her own comfort. Patients with metallic prostheses are not imaged and the operator ensures that no metal is carried into the machine on clothing. The patient does not need to undress. Images are obtained typically in 64 or 128 milliseconds. The slice thickness can be adjusted, but is usually 0.5 or 1 cm. Images are obtained transaxially or coronally.

The patient is placed on the moving bed and pushed into the magnet and pictures taken continuously until the correct plane is found. To obtain the maximum information, patients usually remain in the machine for approximately 20 min, although this could be much shorter if fewer images were required. Approximately 10% of patients complained of mild claustrophobic feelings and in a few cases these were severe enough to necessitate cessation of the study.

Full, informed written consent is always obtained from every patient. Permission for imaging patients within the second or third trimesters of pregnancy has been obtained from the local ethics committee. All of the experiments performed meet the guidelines of the National Radiation Protection Board. All of the fetuses imaged so far have been from pregnancies that have been deemed to be abnormal, with congenital abnormalities or suspected intrauterine growth retardation or problems at the placental site. All but one of the pregnancies (an intrauterine death due to growth retardation 4 weeks after imaging) have proceeded to term and the neonates were (and have remained) healthy. No adverse affects have been recorded by the mothers.

RESULTS

Fetuses have been imaged *in utero* during pregnancies at gestations of between 19 weeks and term. Images have been obtained that clearly show fetal structures including detail of structure within organs. Motional artifact is reduced to a minimum.

Figure 1 shows a sagittal section through a 34-week fetus. This was obtained by taking a coronal section through the mother. The outline of the fetus can clearly be seen looking to the left, facing the placenta. Although features of the face can be seen, the brain appears as a homogeneous mass. Myelination occurs in the fetus late in pregnancy, beginning in the basal ganglia, and therefore the clear differentiation of parts of the brain seen in adults using MRI has, unfortunately, not been available in the obstetric pictures. Using heavily weighted T2 spin sequences it has, however, been possible to obtain some information about the structure of the fetal brain. In the fetal chest the heart can be seen lying anteriorly. The dark areas represent moving blood and in this particular picture the intraventricular septum is clearly seen. Above and posterior to the heart is seen a section through a lung. This appears white with a high signal because it is full of amniotic fluid. The diaphragm is seen as a crisp demarcation between the chest and the abdomen. Loops of bowel are apparent in the abdomen and part of the fetal lower limb can be seen lying in the amniotic fluid which itself has a high signal, conveniently outlining the fetus and the placenta. Figure 2 shows a transaxial section through the chest of a 32-week fetus *in utero*.

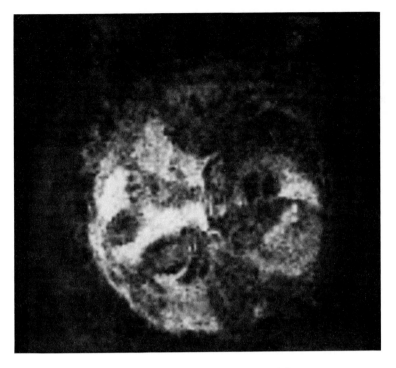

FIG. 1. Sagittal section through a 34-week fetus.

The fetus is lying in the left lower quadrant of the picture surrounded by the white amniotic fluid. The fetus faces its placenta which itself shows a considerable degree of heterogeneity, representing differential blood flow within the organ. The cord can be seen inserting into the placenta. Cross sections through the two fetal arms are also apparent within the amniotic fluid. The organs within the fetal chest are encompassed within a dark ring that on this particular spin sequence represents fetal fat. The fetal heart is seen as a dark area anteriorly within the chest. To either side are the lungs which have a higher signal because of their fluid content. Between the lungs, posteriorly, lies the fetal spinal canal with the CSF showing as a high signal area. Immediately in front of the spinal canal is the vertebral body which is completely dark, in common with other bony tissue.

Figure 3 shows a transaxial section through the upper abdomen of a fetus *in utero* at 37 weeks' gestation. The placenta is seen in the upper portion of the picture running across the anterior wall of the uterus. The fetus lies in the left side of the uterine cavity, the right side being occupied by amniotic fluid with its characteristic high signal. The fetus is facing toward the right side. The high signal area in the midline of the fetal back represents the CSF. Anterolateral to the spinal canal on either side are seen the fetal kidneys with some detail of the calyceal system within each of them. Between the kidneys the rigid ring of the aorta can be seen. Anterior to the left kidney the high signal area is a part of the fluid-filled stomach.

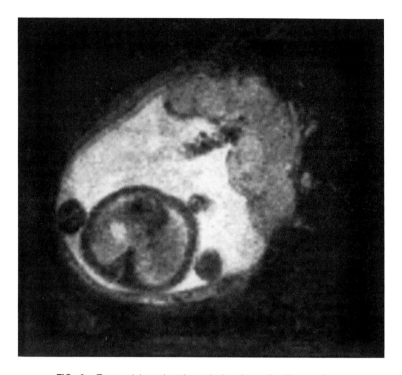

FIG. 2. Transaxial section through the chest of a 32-week fetus.

Figure 4 shows an example of an abnormal fetus imaged using the echo planar technique at 39 weeks' gestation. The placenta covers the anterior wall of the uterine cavity. The fetus lies within the amniotic cavity occupying the right side and facing toward the left. It can be seen that the normal circular abdominal wall is breached anteriorly. Loops of bowel are seen within the amniotic cavity. The extent and size of the defect in the anterior abdominal wall can be estimated.

These are examples of the many images obtained. Approximately 300 such pictures are obtained from every pregnancy imaged.

DISCUSSION

Conventional MRI was first used to image the fetus *in utero* in 1982 by Smith *et al.* (4) and later by Johnson *et al.* (5). Resistive magnets of relatively low strength were used. Image acquisition usually took 2 min or more and although as the fetus became larger more detail became apparent because of the reduction in mobility, the internal structures of the fetus were poorly seen and the technique was disappointing apart from localization of the placenta. Powell *et al.* (6) went on to demonstrate that MRI was superior to ultrasonography in precisely identifying the

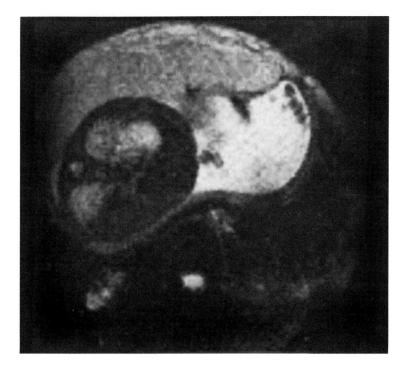

FIG. 3. Transaxial section through the upper abdomen of a 37-week fetus.

placental edge with regard to the internal os of the cervix. Further studies on the fetus, however, even with stronger magnetic fields, were all disappointing. In general only the grossest of fetal abnormalities could be seen. The identification of a fetal organ was regarded as a major triumph, and structure within such an organ was unheard of (7).

Increasing magnet strength has improved resolution and attempts have also been made to reduce image acquisition time using a low flip-angle technique. However, motional artifact is still apparent, and the techniques are of less use in earlier gestations. The number of spin sequences available is also limited. Sedation of the fetus by giving diazepam to the mother may improve the image by reducing fetal motion but this poses ethical problems.

Echo planar imaging, with its ultrashort acquisition time and good resolution, will solve these problems and undoubtedly become the imaging modality technique for obstetrics. At present the technique is in its infancy, but it is clear that pictures of the fetus can be obtained without blurring from motional artifact at gestations in the second and third trimester of pregnancy (8–10). In the structurally normal fetus the development of fetal organs can be studied as pregnancy progresses. Organ volumes can be measured after multiple slice acquisition. Measurement of lung volumes will be of particular importance in cases of suspected lung hypoplasia (for instance in

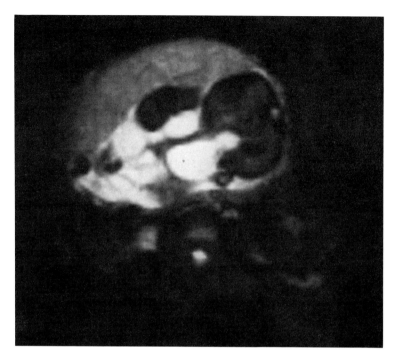

FIG. 4. Transaxial section through the abdomen of a fetus in the 39th week of pregnancy, shows the anterior wall defect of gastroschisis.

severe oligohydramnios). Measurement of liver volume will be of significance in the study of intrauterine growth retardation. The ability to vary the spin sequence used enables us to study fetal fat thickness, again of particular interest in intrauterine growth retardation. Accurate estimation of amniotic fluid volume is simple. In the structurally abnormal fetus EPI is of use in estimating the degree of abnormality, for instance the degree of lung hypoplasia associated with a diaphragmatic hernia.

At present the major difficulty when using EPI is plane selection. Images are taken only in the transverse or coronal plane in relation to the mother. Although this usually gives a transverse or sagittal picture of the fetus, this cannot be guaranteed. Frequently the plane is slightly oblique. These are problems of computer software and will be addressed in time. Because of the expense and relative inconvenience of MRI it will only become an adjunct to ultrasound for particularly difficult cases. The major role of EPI will be in improving the understanding of fetal growth and development, both normal and abnormal. As larger magnets become available (2 tesla and greater) spectroscopy becomes possible. Although spectroscopy is currently performed using conventional MRI, the combination of the speed of signal acquisition using EPI and spectroscopy will be of particular value in studying fetal biochemistry. EPI is the obstetricians research tool of the future.

REFERENCES

1. Mansfield P. Multiplanar image formation using NMR spin echoes. *J Physics c: Solid State Physics* 1977;10:L55–8.
2. Mansfield P, Pikett IL. Biological and medical imaging by NMR. *J Magn Reson* 1978;29:355–73.
3. Chapman B, Turner R, Ordidge RJ, *et al.* Real-time movie imaging from a single cardiac cycle by NMR. *Magn Reson Med* 1987;5:246–54.
4. Smith FW, McClennan F, Abramovitch DR, McGillavry I, Hutchison JMS. NMR imaging in human pregnancy: a preliminary study. *Magn Reson Imaging* 1984;2:57–64.
5. Johnson IR, Symonds EM, Kean DM, *et al.* Imaging the pregnant human uterus with nuclear magnetic resonance. *Am J Obstet Gynecol* 1984;148:1136–9.
6. Powell MC, Buckley J, Symonds EM, Worthington BS. Magnetic resonance imaging and placenta praevia. *Am J Obstet Gynecol* 1986;154:565–9.
7. Weinreb JC, Lowe T, Curran JM, Kutler M. Human fetal anatomy: MR Imaging. *Radiology* 1985;159:715–20.
8. Johnson IR, Stehling MK, Blamire AM, *et al.* Study of internal structure of the human uterus in utero by echo planar magnetic resonance imaging. *Am J Obstet Gynecol* 1990;63:833–41.
9. Stehling MK, Mansfield P, Ordidge RJ, *et al.* Echo planar magnetic resonance imaging in abnormal pregnancies. *Lancet* 1989;2:157–8.
10. Stehling MK, Mansfield P, Ordidge RJ, *et al.* Echo planar imaging of the human fetus in utero. *Magn Reson Med* 1990;13:314–8.

DISCUSSION

Dr. Fujiwara: What is the earliest gestational age at which you can identify spina bifida?

Dr. Johnson: Identification of spina bifida with MRI depends on the plane in which the fetus is seen. If you happen to view the spine in the sagittal plane you will identify spina bifida very easily and be able to identify its exact extent, but you may not be able to guarantee that the fetus does not have spina bifida if the viewing angle is not ideal. The earliest fetuses we have looked at were 16 weeks, when a reasonable amount of detail can be seen. In the first trimester it is not very easy to see anything. Ultrasound is vastly superior at this stage.

Dr. Fujiwara: So many cases of spina bifida have a miserable outcome that perhaps the development of mass screening should be considered.

Dr. Johnson: Mass screening already exists. I can't remember having seen a spina bifida patient at term in the last 2 to 3 years. Alpha-fetoprotein screening is as near 100% as we can make it in our particular region. We also feel that it is ethical to perform ultrasound routinely on every patient, and many of the larger hospitals are doing this at 17 or 18 weeks. I think we are picking up most neural tube defects in this way.

Dr. Hope: Is there any danger to the fetus from the noise made by MRI?

Dr. Johnson: I'm not sure about this. I have been trying to think how we could measure it. As the fetus is effectively under water I think it hears less noise than the mother.

Dr. Hope: Are there paramagnetic agents that would pass across the placenta and aid in visualizing the fetal heart or kidney?

Dr. Johnson: We haven't considered them yet. I don't know about placental transfer of paramagnetic agents. There are so many problems about the ethics of imaging patients in pregnancy without yet further degrees of intervention that I feel this is an area that we should not venture into at present. In fact we avoid using conventional MRI to view the fetus for these reasons.

Dr. Schmidt: Do you think it would be possible to obtain more information about the lungs with your techniques? I am especially interested in biophysical and biochemical information about the lung, phospholipids, relaxation times, and so on.

Dr. Johnson: I do not have very much data in this area at present. We have just started experiments where in addition to looking at lung volume we try to use different spin sequences, particularly from 16 weeks on, to see if we can identify a change in the chemical nature of the lung as it matures. Clearly it would be of major clinical benefit if you could take a picture of the fetus at 32 weeks and decide how mature the lungs were. I am reasonably optimistic about our chances of being able to do this because there must be considerable chemical changes in the phospholipids that we should be able to recognize.

Dr. Saling: Do you think it will be possible in the future to differentiate between lung hypoplasia caused by lack of amniotic fluid and normal lung tissue.

Dr. Johnson: There may be chemical differences in hypoplastic lung compared with normal lung that could be demonstrated using different spin sequences, but it will take a long time to acquire this information because of the difficulty in finding enough fetuses with hypoplastic lungs to image. As far as lung volume is concerned, I think that when we have established the normal volume pattern during different stages of gestation it will be possible to identify the underdeveloped lung. In one case of diaphragmatic hernia that we studied it was possible to see clearly how compressed and underdeveloped in volume terms the lungs were.

Dr. Van Geijn: Six or seven years ago I heard some work from Berlin in which it was shown that there was a very nice correlation between lactic acid and NDPH in guinea pig brain. There was a promise that before long it would be possible to measure lactic acid phosphate rate compounds in the human brain, which would have important implications for obstetrics. Why don't we have these data by now?

Dr. Johnson: I think the reason is mainly technical. We can't get these data because our magnet is only 0.5 tesla and to perform spectroscopy you need a 1.5 or 2 tesla magnet. There are units with stronger magnets. The unit in Liverpool for example is doing spectroscopy on their 2 tesla magnet, but only on the placenta. I suspect the reason for not studying the fetus is that they have found it impossible to look with any reliability at the same part of the fetus repeatedly. I think that eventually a combination of fast imaging technique and spectroscopy will get over this problem.

As far as lactate is concerned the problem is that because of the number of neutrons and protons you can't actually look at the carbon, so you can't look at lactate directly.

Dr. Hope: Spatially localized spectroscopy on a moving target is very difficult. Signal-to-noise ratio is very low once you are looking deeper than 5 cm, and will be aggravated by movement. Lactate can be studied using high-resolution proton spectroscopy and special techniques to suppress the huge signal from water. We have used this technique in animals, as have many other groups, but it will be very difficult to apply to a moving target at a considerable distance.

Perinatology, edited by Erich Saling,
Nestlé Nutrition Workshop Series, Vol. 26,
Nestec, Ltd., Vevey/Raven Press, Ltd.,
New York © 1992.

Recent Progress in Prenatal Ultrasonic Diagnosis

Pentti Jouppila

Department of Obstetrics and Gynecology, University of Oulu, 90220 Oulu, Finland

The use of diagnostic ultrasound in obstetrics started in the late 1960s and became universally accepted over the next 10 years. Its rapid technical and methodological development has gone from the initial one- and two-dimensional black-and-white images to gray-scale techniques, and then to the real-time method, enabling the dynamic demonstration of different intrauterine objects. During the 1980s the introduction of Doppler and recently the color Doppler techniques has opened up diagnostic possibilities for the examination of fetal hemodynamics and cardiac function. During this 20-year period the resolution capacity of ultrasonic equipment has been markedly improved and so the detailed examination of the fetal organs and tissues is often reliable as early as the late first and early second trimester of pregnancy.

The evaluation of progress in diagnostic ultrasound in prenatal medicine depends on the particular focus of interest. The following areas have been at the forefront of development and further progress in these fields is to be expected in the future:

1. Comprehensive diagnosis and increased knowledge of fetal anomalies and congenital syndromes
2. Transvaginal ultrasound
3. Invasive measures performed by ultrasonic guidance
4. Doppler and color Doppler methods.

In all of these fields development has led to increased anatomic and physiologic knowledge and also to improvements in daily obstetric practice. Even so, the techniques pose new diagnostic problems that will need intensive research in the near future.

FETAL ANOMALIES

In nearly all the leading obstetric journals case reports dealing with "new" fetal abnormalities have appeared during the last few years. This is due to the wide use of diagnostic ultrasound in everyday obstetrics. It is, however, of more importance

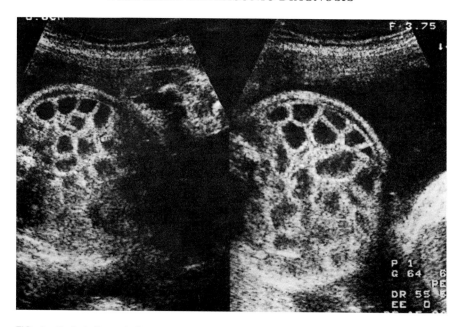

FIG. 1. Typical ultrasonic finding of fluid-filled bowels in congenital chloride diarrhea. Twin pregnancy, both fetuses are affected.

that the whole picture of the anomaly spectrum has been clarified. Hence the detection of one fetal abnormality is very often combined with the identification of some specific syndrome or chromosomal aberration, or with a hereditary background. In investigating these conditions cooperation between pediatricians, clinical geneticists, and pathologists is very important. An example of the early prenatal ultrasonic diagnosis of single-gene diseases with a specific pattern of inheritance is congenital chloride diarrhea, in which fluid-filled bowel structures can be seen as a typical ultrasonic finding in the fetal abdominal cavity (Fig. 1). In lethal congenital contracture syndrome the early appearance of fetal hydrops and lack of fetal movements are the typical findings. Most of the structural fetal abnormalities are primarily found or suspected in ultrasound screening procedures or in examinations made for other reasons. However, the indications for a thorough ultrasonic evaluation of the fetal anatomy have been specified during the last few years. They include:

1. Anamnestic warning: maternal autoimmune diseases, specific drugs, etc.
2. Fetal hydrops
3. Early growth retardation
4. Oligo- or polyhydramnion
5. Lack of fetal movements
6. Heart arrhythmias
7. Placental hydrops and multiple cysts.

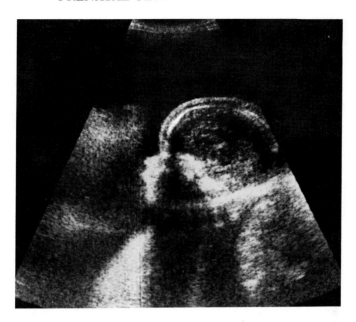

FIG. 2. Fetal hydrops demonstrated as a separation of skull bone and skin contours.

Interpretation of the ultrasonic findings and their prognostic evaluation needs great experience and so suspected cases should be referred to second- or third-level clinics. Also the ability to determine fetal chromosomal status by blood sampling, placental biopsy, or amniocentesis must be available in these centers.

An illustrative example of the diagnostic problems connected with fetal abnormalities is fetal hydrops (Fig. 2). It is well known that there are many etiological factors in this condition. Cardiovascular defects or diseases can be found in nearly 25%, chromosomal abnormalities in 10%, and fetal infections in 5%. So the ultrasonic finding on its own does not help in the further diagnostic and prognostic evaluation of the affected fetus. On the other hand, the spontaneous resolution of hydrops is not a rare observation and justifies careful follow-up of the affected cases. The severe forms of hydrops often occur in the final stages of fetal disease and the prognosis is likely to be bad regardless of the type of intervention. The criteria and selection of hydropic fetuses for nonactive or active follow-up or treatment needs the availability of fetal blood sampling and the ability to undertake specific examination of heart structures. Another example of the prognostic problems posed by new techniques is the significance of choroid plexus cysts diagnosed by ultrasound in fetal brains in the second trimester (Fig. 3). Most small unilateral cysts seem to disappear between weeks 20 and 24 but choroid plexus cysts are, on the other hand, common in trisomy 18, suggesting that there should be further evaluation of fetal structures and consideration of chromosome analysis (1). The setting of exact indications for

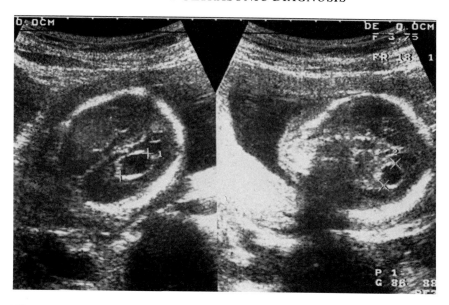

FIG. 3. Unilateral choroid plexus cyst in the fetal brain at the 24th week. Two ultrasonic sections.

invasive procedures in individual cases is difficult, as is communicating these issues to the parents.

Examples of prognostically bad ultrasonic findings in connection with fetal structural abnormalities are the occurrence of multiple anomalies and the early development of poly- or oligohydramnios and fetal hydrops. On the other hand, an unpredictable course is common in early fetal hydronephrosis (Fig. 4), fetal arrhythmias, and milder forms of fetal pleural effusion and ascites. In female fetuses regular cystic formations in the pelvis, outside the urinary tract, are often ovarian cysts which usually have no harmful effects on the function of neighboring organs.

The recent challenges in the diagnosis of fetal anomalies are more and more concentrating on examination of the functional capacity of the affected organs (brain, kidney, heart, etc.), especially in attempting to select between active and nonactive follow-up of pregnancy and the timing of delivery. The search for associated anomalies and for chromosomal abnormalities must be included in the further and prognostic evaluation of, for example, kidney, heart, and central nervous system anomalies. One prognostic problem is presented by fetal abdominal space-occupying lesions, which can markedly affect and compress the lungs so that the alveoli are not able to open after delivery. The contours of the fetal face and the detailed examination of the distal parts of the limbs (Fig. 5) are examples of the possibilities of modern ultrasonic prenatal diagnosis. Abnormal findings such as micrognathia and abnormal number of fingers can give warning signals for fetal trisomies or some specific hereditary syndromes. It is evident, however, that the final conclusions to be based on such findings must be the prerogative of high-level centers.

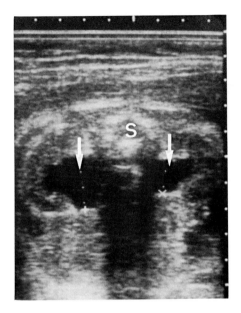

FIG. 4. Bilateral enlargement of fetal kidney pelvis (*arrows*). Ultrasonic cross section. S, spine.

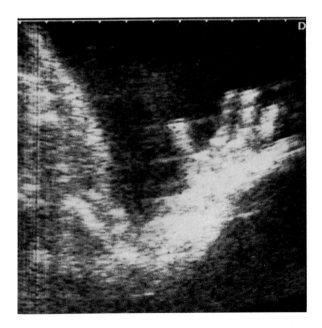

FIG. 5. Fetal hand and fingers demonstrated by ultrasound. Normal finding.

TRANSVAGINAL ULTRASOUND

The introduction of special probes for transvaginal examinations has opened some new avenues for ultrasonic studies, especially during early pregnancy. The benefits are based on the short distance between probe and target organs, leading to the use of higher frequencies in the probes (5–7 mHz), which enables the better resolution of the tissues. There is no need for a full-bladder technique, which shortens the total time needed for the examination. The essential findings in early pregnancy, such as the gestation sac, the embryo, and signs of viability can be detected about one week earlier than with the transabdominal technique. Some fetal anomalies can be found as early as the last few weeks of the first trimester of pregnancy. It must also be stressed that in the later stages of pregnancy the structural evaluation of the presenting part of fetal body can be made in more detail by this route. The proper evaluation of the cervix in threatening premature delivery, of the isthmic region in repeated cesarean sections, and of the exact correlation between the placental margin and the cervical internal os can also be made using transvaginal probes. The greatest practical benefit of this technique has obviously been in the improved and earlier detection of ectopic pregnancies.

In this area there are also many practical problems. When examining the embryonal structures during the organogenetic stage the borderline between normal and abnormal findings can be very unclear, for example the fetal abdominal organs around the 10th week of pregnancy are partly outside the abdominal cavity, mimicking umbilical hernia. Nomograms dealing with early fetal biometry are largely lacking. So in cases of suspected anomaly serial follow-up studies are necessary.

INVASIVE PRENATAL MEASURES PERFORMED BY ULTRASONIC GUIDANCE

Oocyte retrieval *in vitro* fertilization (IVF) programs is chronologically the first step in the various types of instrumentation made under ultrasonic supervision in relation to pregnancy. This transvaginal puncture has totally replaced the earlier laparoscopic methods. Chorion villous sampling either transvaginally or transabdominally guided by ultrasound, is also in routine use for the analysis of fetal chromosome and DNA structures at the 8th through 12th weeks of pregnancy. Early amniocentesis during these weeks is also possible from a methodological ultrasonic point of view. Extraction of an IUD during the first trimester of pregnancy is reasonable due to the 40 to 50% threat of late abortion or very premature delivery if the device is left in the uterus. If the tails cannot be seen in the cervix, removal is still possible using special forceps under ultrasonic guidance.

Transvaginal aspiration of multiple gestational sacs can be considered in IVF pregnancies with more than three or four sacs. This procedure is possible using ultrasonic supervision. There are also possibilities for the early transvaginal salpingocentesis of unruptured tubal pregnancies under ultrasonic guidance (2), which could be one

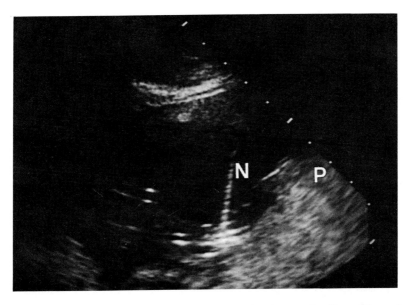

FIG. 6. Fetal blood sampling from the umbilical vessels by ultrasound guidance. N, needle: P, placenta.

possibility in the development of more conservative approaches to the treatment of ectopic pregnancy.

Fetal blood sampling from the umbilical vessels, which is possible transabdominally under ultrasound guidance, is obviously one of the greatest achievements of modern diagnostic obstetrics. A 20 to 23 G needle is directed transamniotically, and sometimes transplacentally, to the umbilical vein or artery. The place of choice is the placental insertion of the cord, which is the most stabile place for needling (Fig. 6). The other potential targets for blood sampling are the intra-abdominal part of fetal umbilical vein or the fetal heart. Direct sampling of fetal blood allows the estimation of many variables as in adults (acid-base balance, infectious agents, chromosomes, etc.). The answers reflect fetal physiological or biochemical status directly instead of indirectly, as is the case with amniotic fluid analysis. These rapid direct answers are of great help in the practical management of many obstetric problems. Fetal blood sampling has brought a new understanding of fetal pathophysiology in conditions such as chronic fetal distress and hemolytic disease. The detection of new fetal diseases is theoretically possible by this technique.

The central indications for fetal blood sampling include:

1. Suspicion of fetal chromosomal abnormality (structural anomalies known to be associated with cytogenetic pathology, early growth retardation, etc.)
2. Chronic fetal asphyxia suspected after noninvasive investigations
3. Severe Rh-isoimmunization
4. Nonimmunologic fetal hydrops

5. Suspicion of fetal infection
6. Maternal severe thrombocytopenia (alloimmune form)
7. Suspicion of twin-to-twin or fetomaternal transfusion
8. Hemoglobinopathies.

One example of the new knowledge obtained by this technique is an understanding of the normal distribution of fetal hemoglobin levels during the second half of pregnancy. Using this knowledge in cases of severe Rh-isoimmunization, umbilical blood sampling gives rapid information about the actual degree of hemolysis (3). The sampling can be immediately followed by blood transfusion if necessary, given into an umbilical vessel. Correspondingly the pH, pO_2, and lactate levels can be determined in suspected fetal asphyxia and the values can be compared with normal values, thus helping the obstetrical decision making (3).

The potential side effects of fetal blood sampling are the following:

1. Bleeding from the punctured umbilical vessel. This continues for more than 1 min in only 1–5%. Exsanguination has not been observed.
2. Fetal bradycardia in 5–10%, with normalization in 1–2 min.
3. Fetomaternal bleeding. This may exacerbate the severity of Rh-isoimmunization.
4. Chorionamnionitis and premature rupture of the membranes are possible but very rare complications.
5. Immediate fetal death, possibly associated with blood tamponade of the umbilical cord. The number of fetal deaths is universally associated with the indication for sampling. Frequency in large series is 0.5–1%.

Fetal blood sampling is a procedure that, in addition to good ultrasonic equipment and technical skills, also requires a sufficient number of cases and its regular use to minimize the occurrence of side effects. It should be concentrated in clinics with a particular experience of the technique. Many problems await solutions, such as the optimal intervals and the safety of repeated sampling.

DOPPLER AND COLOR DOPPLER METHODS

Until the late 1970s the only methods by which data on uteroplacental and fetal hemodynamics could be obtained were chronic animal models, utilizing electromagnetic probes or radiolabeled microspheres, and isotope methods in human studies. During the last 10 years the introduction of combined real-time and Doppler techniques, supplemented recently by color Doppler, has made possible the examination of hemodynamics in fetal and uterine vessels. Totally new knowledge of fetal physiology has been obtained, helping our understanding of fetal adaptative processes, for example chronic asphyxia. As a noninvasive and safe method the Doppler technique can today be utilized in combination with other methods in obstetric practice.

Methodological difficulties that affect the reliability of volume blood flow studies have shifted practical interest to special indices of the arterial blood velocity

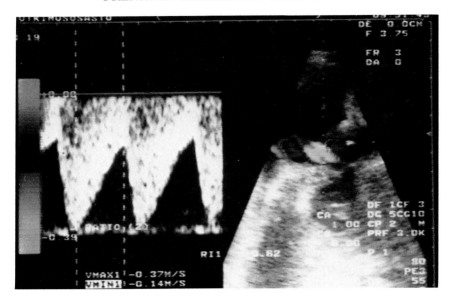

FIG. 7. Demonstration of the location of umbilical coiled vessels and the normal blood velocity waveform from the umbilical artery (colors unfortunately cannot be demonstrated in this and the following figures for printing reasons).

waveforms: pulsatility index (PI), resistance index (RI), and systolic/diastolic ratio (S/D). These parameters are dependent on many regulators such as cardiac contraction forces and pulse frequency, but particularly on the peripheral vascular resistance distal to the point of measurement. This theoretical background has been documented in many studies. Trudinger *et al.* (4) have demonstrated, for example, that embolization of the umbilical arteries of fetal sheep significantly raised the index values of these vessels measured by the Doppler method. The vessel count in small villi also showed a significant negative correlation with the S/D ratio of umbilical arteries (5).

Regulation of fetal hemodynamics is mainly determined by the oxygen demands of fetal tissues. Low peripheral vascular resistance is typical in both the uterine and the main fetal arteries (umbilical artery, descending aorta). Hemodynamic redistribution in favor of the cerebral circulation, which has earlier been demonstrated in animal models during chronic hypoxia, has also been clearly documented in the human fetal circulation. The obvious primary background of this change is the narrowing process of the small maternal uteroplacental and fetal villous vessels in hypertensive diseases leading to an increase in placental vascular resistance.

The main vessel and the first to be studied in clinical practice is the umbilical artery. Flow indices decline throughout normal pregnancy, and after the 16th week there are always detectable end-diastolic frequencies (Fig. 7). The indices increase in chronic fetal asphyxia above the normal range. Absent end-diastolic velocity in the umbilical artery or in the descending aorta predicts with a sensitivity of 70–80%

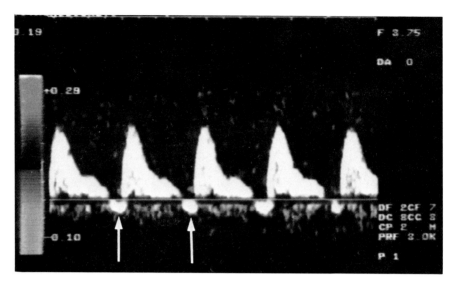

FIG. 8. Reverse end-diastolic flow (*arrows*) in the umbilical artery blood velocity waveform in fetal asphyxia.

the perinatal signs of chronic asphyxia (cesarean section for chronic fetal distress, need for admission to neonatal intensive care unit, perinatal mortality)(6). It is important to stress that a methodologically false finding of absent end-diastolic velocity can be obtained if the filter level in the Doppler equipment is over 150 Hz or if the angle between the vessel and Doppler beam approaches 90°. The even more pathologic finding (reverse end-diastolic flow) (Fig. 8) in the umbilical artery predicts perinatal mortality in 50–100% (7). On the other hand, the sensitivity in identifying SGA fetuses (weight under the 10th percentile of normal range) varies between 30% and 50% in different series (8,9). This relatively low sensitivity is mainly based on the fact that many genetically small but well-being fetuses are included in this group and umbilical velocity waveforms are quite normal in these cases. Although most of the pathologic waveforms in the umbilical artery occur in cases of chronic asphyxia these findings can also occur in fetal structural or chromosomal abnormalities in approximately 50% (10). So the exact evaluation of fetal anatomy by ultrasound and the potential use of chromosome analysis must be considered in these cases.

The second vessel of interest in clinical practice is the main branch of the uterine artery. Originally the arterial velocity waveforms were registered from the small myometrial vessels, arcuate arteries, by using continuous-wave Doppler but methodological inaccuracies leading to high variability of index values in the arcuate arteries have focused the studies into the main uterine arteries. Color Doppler has markedly improved the localization of these vessels and their differentation from the other neighboring arteries (Fig. 9). A rapid fall in flow indices in the uterine arteries can be detected at 13 to 20 weeks followed by a more gentle fall thereafter. This

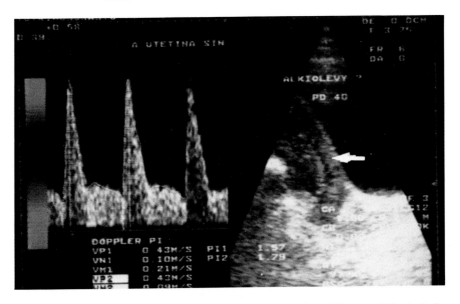

FIG. 9. Demonstration of the uterine artery (*arrow*) by color Doppler and the normal blood velocity waveform of this vessel during the late second trimester of pregnancy.

suggests decreasing vascular resistance in the peripheral spiral arteries. A notch (Fig. 10) in early diastole, a sign of high peripheral vascular resistance, must have disappeared by 24 to 26 weeks. Lack of decrease in indices or persistence of this notch is predictive (sensitivity 40–50%) of the development of pre-eclampsia, intrauterine growth retardation, and fetal asphyxia in late pregnancy (11), though conflicting results have been obtained (12) demonstrating that this kind of correlation may not be ready as a screening test. Methodologically important is the observation that the site of the placenta affects the velocity waveforms of the two uterine arteries (13). It is probable that flow studies of uterine arteries are preferable until the 24th through 26th week, and umbilical and fetal arterial examination thereafter. The waveforms of the uterine arteries also seem to react more sensitively to different maternal vasoactive agents (antihypertensive or tocolytic drugs, epidural anesthesia) compared to the umbilical arteries (14). The differentiation between the placental and the myometrial circulation is not yet possible by Doppler studies of the uterine arteries. According to animal studies many antihypertensive drugs dilate only the myometrial arteries and have vasoconstrictor effects on the placental circulation (15).

In normal pregnancies the end-diastolic blood velocity in the fetal cerebral arteries is lower than that in, for example, the umbilical artery but end-diastolic blood flow is always present during the third trimester. The vessels of main interest are the middle cerebral arteries, which can easily be identified by color Doppler (Fig. 11) and very often also by the usual pulsed Doppler, and the common or internal carotid arteries. Flow indices in these arteries fall after the 32nd through 34th week suggesting the centralization of the blood flow toward term also in nonhypoxemic

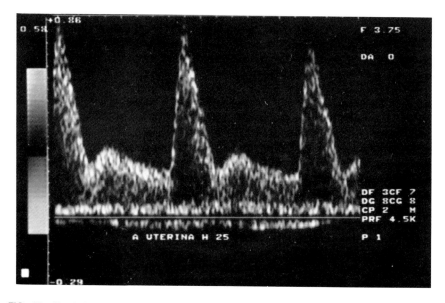

FIG. 10. Notch finding in the early diastole in the uterine artery blood velocity waveform at the 30th week of pregnancy in a case of severe intrauterine growth retardation.

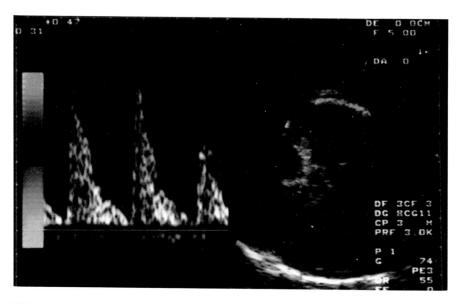

FIG. 11. Location of the fetal middle cerebral artery by color Doppler and its normal blood velocity waveform.

fetuses. Decreased vascular resistance with low indices is a typical consequence of chronic fetal asphyxia and has been clearly demonstrated in human fetuses (16). It is, however, still unclear how much the recording of carotid or cerebral blood velocity waveforms can help or improve diagnostic conclusions made on the basis of studies of uterine and umbilical arteries alone.

In conclusion it can be said that the use of the Doppler method in trained hands is suitable for clinical obstetric practice. Its main value is the differentiation between the chronically asphyxiated fetus from the small healthy fetus. Pathologic findings in umbilical and uterine arteries give an early and relatively sensitive warning signal of chronic fetal asphyxia preceding other signs such as those obtained by cardiotocography by several days or even weeks (17). We still have no clear clinical concept of the meaning of pathologic Doppler findings. Fetal capacity to tolerate a pathologic or redistributed circulation seems to be variable. In some cases the umbilical blood acid-base value shows normal levels at a time of clearly pathologic blood velocity waveforms in the umbilical artery (18). So the timing of delivery cannot be based on the Doppler findings alone, but must depend as well on all the additional "traditional" methods (clinical evaluation, ultrasound for elucidation of fetal size and structures, biophysical scoring, and fetal blood samples). In many cases the timing of delivery remains a compromise between threatening fetal asphyxia and prematurity, because adverse changes in hemodynamics have often already begun during the late second trimester of pregnancy. Although the first randomized studies have shown beneficial effects when Doppler methods have been used in the surveillance of selected pathologic pregnancies (19), it is still difficult to assess whether the Doppler technique can improve the perinatal results obtained using earlier methods in developed countries. The major current challenges in this new diagnostic area are in studies of small peripheral fetal arteries (kidney, iliac, femoral) and in the search and critical assessment of the methods focusing on attempts to treat chronic fetal asphyxia.

REFERENCES

1. Fitzsimmons J, Wilson D, Pascoe-Mason J, *et al.* Choroid plexus cysts in fetuses with trisomy 18. *Obstet Gynecol* 1989;73:257–60.
2. Timor-Tritsch I, Baxi L, Peisner DB. Transvaginal salpingocentesis: a new technique for treating ectopic pregnancy. *Am J Obstet Gynecol* 1980;160:459–61.
3. Soothill PW. Cordocentesis: role in assessment of fetal condition. *Clin Perinatol* 1989;16:755–70.
4. Trudinger BJ, Stevens D, Connelly A, *et al.* Umbilical artery flow velocity waveforms and placental resistance: the effects of embolization of the umbilical circulation. *Am J Obstet Gynecol* 1987;157:1143–8.
5. Giles WB, Trudinger BJ, Baird PJ. Fetal umbilical artery flow velocity waveforms and placental resistance: pathological correlation. *Br J Obstet Gynaecol* 1985;92:31–8.
6. Jouppila P, Kirkinen P. Noninvasive assessment of fetal aortic blood flow in normal and abnormal pregnancies. *Clin Obstet Gynecol* 1989;32:703–9.
7. Brar HS, Platt LD. Reverse end-diastolic flow velocity on umbilical artery velocimetry in high-risk pregnancies: an ominous finding with adverse pregnancy outcome. *Am J Obstet Gynecol* 1988;159:559–61.
8. Berkowitz GS, Chitkara U, Rosenberg J, *et al.* Sonographic estimation of fetal weight and Doppler

analysis of umbilical artery velocimetry in the prediction of intrauterine growth retardation: a prospective study. *Am J Obstet Gynecol* 1988;158:1149–53.

9. Beattie RB, Dornan JG. Antenatal screening for intrauterine growth retardation with umbilical artery Doppler ultrasonography. *Br Med J* 1989;298:631–5.

10. Trudinger BJ, Cook CM. Umbilical and uterine artery flow velocity waveforms in pregnancy associated with major fetal abnormality. *Br J Obstet Gynaecol* 1985;92:666–70.

11. Arduini D, Rizzo G, Romanini C, et al. Uteroplacental flow velocity waveforms as predictors of pregnancy-induced hypertension. *Eur J Obstet Gynecol Reprod Biol* 1987;26:335–41.

12. Jacobsson SL, Imhof R, Manning R, et al. The value of Doppler assessment of the uteroplacental circulation in predicting pre-eclampsia or intrauterine growth retardation. *Am J Obstet Gynecol* 1990;162:110–4.

13. Kofinas AD, Penry M, Greiss FC, et al. The effect of placental location on uterine artery flow velocity waveforms. *Am J Obstet Gynecol* 1988;159:1504–8.

14. Pirhonen JP, Erkkola RU, Ekblad UU. Uterine and fetal flow velocity waveforms in hypertensive pregnancy: the effect of a single dose of nifedipine. *Obstet Gynecol* 1990;76:37–41.

15. Parisi VM, Rankin JHG. The effect of prostacyclin on angiotensin II–induced placental vasoconstriction. *Am J Obstet Gynecol* 1985;151:444–9.

16. Wladimiroff JW, Noordam MJ, van den Wijngaard JAG, et al. Cerebral and umbilical arterial blood flow velocity waveforms in normal and growth retarded pregnancies: a comparative study. *Obstet Gynecol* 1987;69:705–9.

17. Jouppila P. Doppler findings in the fetal and uteroplacental circulation: a promising guide to clinical decisions. *Ann Med* 1990;22:109–13.

18. Nicolaides KH, Bilardo CM, Soothill PV, et al. Absence of end-diastolic frequencies in umbilical artery: a sign of fetal hypoxia and acidosis. *Br Med J* 1988;297:1026–7.

19. Trudinger BJ, Cook CM, Giles WB, et al. Umbilical artery flow velocity waveforms in high-risk pregnancy trial. *Lancet* 1987;1:188–90.

DISCUSSION

Dr. Van Geijn: There is debate about whether reversed flow in the fetal aorta is due to increased resistance in the placental bed or to a reduction in flow. From your series of cases with reversed flow, do you have data on umbilical, carotid, and renal artery blood flow, and could you comment on what is the most likely cause of this reversed flow in the fetal aorta?

Dr. Jouppila: Most of the flow in the descending aorta goes to the umbilical artery, so it is common to find the same pathologic findings in these two vessels. I believe that in most cases the reversal of flow in the descending aorta is due more to increased resistance in the umbilical-placental circulation than to that in fetal peripheral arteries, but I have no personal data to prove this.

Dr. Gold: Can you give further detail about the relationship between blood flow disturbances and chromosomal abnormalities? In my town in France, they don't believe this relationship exists and won't do karyotyping when they find blood flow abnormalities, even though some teams in Paris have shown what you describe.

Dr. Jouppila: It is very important to consider fetal abnormalities when we have pathologic findings in fetal hemodynamics. Wladimiroff has observed that if the fetus has a chromosomal abnormality, the centralization or decreased resistance in cerebral arteries, a common finding in otherwise normal fetuses with intrauterine growth retardation (IUGR) is absent. In our own studies we have data from five or six cases with anomalies and the situation is not so clear-cut. We have found centralization of the fetal circulation in the middle cerebral arteries to be present in some cases of chromosomal abnormality and not in others. I am not entirely certain how we can separate chromosomal abnormalities from normal IUGR by the hemodynamic findings.

Dr. Kurjak: There are two different types of IUGR that should be differentiated prenatally. In symmetrical growth retardation there is a strong association with chromosomal abnormalities and a low growth potential. There is no evidence of hypoxia. Asymmetrically growth-retarded babies have evidence of placental insufficiency, and in a significant proportion we can detect perinatal asphyxia. Thus before we draw any conclusions about how abnormal Doppler measurements can differentiate between chromosomally normal and chromosomally abnormal growth-retarded babies, let us do biometry and distinguish the type of growth retardation as early as possible.

Dr. Eschenbach: Certain hypotensive states in the mother are associated with very high maternal cardiac output. Have you had a chance to follow fetal blood flow in these individuals?

Dr. Jouppila: Huch's group in Switzerland has made such comparative studies. Fetal blood flow seems to adapt to changes in maternal hemodynamics very well.

Dr. Kurjak: This is a good comment. Whatever happens in fetal blood flow is a result of pathology elsewhere. Thus we need to study maternal blood flow. Is it still difficult to locate the uterine arteries using color Doppler?

Dr. Jouppila: The main problem is in locating the smaller arcuate vessels, rather than the main uterine arteries. We cannot always be sure we are looking at the same vessel. Sometimes also the main uterine artery may have a delta of divisions before entering the uterine wall, so it may be hard to know which branch to measure. Although color Doppler has made identification much easier we still have problems.

Dr. Dawes: I have read suggestions that flow velocity waveform measurements made in the two umbilical arteries differ. One can see how this could happen if there is an infarct in an area of the placenta fed by one umbilical artery. In your experience has this ever occurred? Do you regularly look at both umbilical arteries?

Dr. Jouppila: If there are clearly different findings in the two umbilical arteries, the first possibility in my opinion is methodological error. In many cases, when using indices, it may be impossible to determine the exact angle at which the vessel is being viewed, and the angle can be quite different for the two vessels. If the angle is near 90°, end-diastolic velocity may be lost. This is the main explanation, but there are other possibilities. Trudinger has published a case report in which there were clearly different index values in the two umbilical arteries. After birth it was found that a part of the placenta was infarcted. Another possibility is failure to recognize the fact that indices are lower if umbilical artery waveforms are measured near the placental insertion than they are near the fetal insertion.

Dr. Dawes: Resistance indices taken by the same individual on the same patient may be quite variable from day to day. Is this your experience?

Dr. Jouppila: We do not get very great intra- and interexaminer variability. I feel that training is most important in avoiding such methodological problems. However my opinion is that in clinical practice we must put our trust in the visual findings and not rely too heavily on indices. The absent end-diastolic velocity in the umbilical artery is a really pathological finding, and we are sure that the methodology is satisfactory in identifying this.

Dr. Dawes: The truth is that it is somebody's observation. When someone tells me there is no end-diastolic flow this is an opinion based on visual analysis. There may be an error of 15–20%. If you are going to take action on such findings, the measurements should be repeated several times. What is your clinical practice?

Dr. Jouppila: We do not make clinical decisions solely on these findings. We follow the patients very closely. If we know that we have identified absent end-diastolic velocity, we use all possible monitoring systems. But at 26 to 28 weeks, for example, we cannot make decisions based on Doppler findings alone.

Dr. Saling: From a clinical point of view, and recalling how many cesarean sections have been performed on the basis only of some suspicion about the cardiotocogram, then having this method available is certainly an advance, irrespective of its sources of inaccuracy.

Perinatology, edited by Erich Saling,
Nestlé Nutrition Workshop Series, Vol. 26,
Nestec, Ltd., Vevey/Raven Press, Ltd.,
New York © 1992.

How Objective is Visual Evaluation of Antepartum and Intrapartum Cardiotocograms?

Herman P. Van Geijn, *Dick K. Donker, and *Arie Hasman

*Department of Obstetrics and Gynecology, Free University Hospital, De Boelelaan 1117, P.O. Box 7057, 1007 MB Amsterdam, The Netherlands; and *Department of Medical Informatics and Statistics, University of Limburg, P.B. Box 616, 6200 MD Maastricht, The Netherlands*

Decisions to intervene during pregnancy or labor because of fetal distress can be determined by many factors such as maternal hypertension, fetal growth retardation, a decrease in fetal movements, a diminished amount of amniotic fluid, an abnormal blood flow in fetal or umbilical vessels, and an abnormal fetal heart rate pattern. The final decision to actually perform a cesarean section (in pregnancy or labor) or a forceps or ventouse delivery (in labor) is still in the majority of cases based upon the heart rate pattern recorded from the fetus.

Fetal heart rate (FHR) as a sign of fetal well-being was at first recognized around 1820. Until the years 1965 to 1970, intermittent auscultation using a stethoscope was the only method available. Electronic monitoring of FHR and maternal uterine activity (cardiotocography) was then introduced by Caldeyro-Barcia *et al.* (1), Hon and Quilligan (2), and Hammacher (3) at approximately the same time in South America, the United States, and Europe, respectively.

Continuous monitoring of FHR, in comparison with intermittent auscultation, is now easily performed, provides accurate and continuous information, and results in a substantial document. It is relatively cheap compared with other surveillance techniques. Cardiotocographic monitoring is used in at-risk pregnancies, for example 30 to 60 min several times per week or on a daily basis. During labor it is applied for a longer period and often continuously during the major part of the first and second stage of labor.

Signs of fetal distress include tachycardia (baseline FHR more than 160 beats/min), bradycardia (baseline FHR less than 100 beats/min), diminished or absent variability, absence of accelerations for more than 40 min, and presence of decelerations either spontaneously, during movements of the fetus, or in relation to uterine contractions (4). Particularly variable and late decelerations are associated with a lowering of fetal pH. Increasing duration and depth of decelerations and shortening of pauses between decelerations are among the factors that lead the obstetrician to believe that fetal condition is deteriorating (5).

67

VALIDITY OF CARDIOTOCOGRAPHY

Although techniques of electronic fetal heart rate monitoring (EFM) have improved in the last decades, the validity of cardiotocography remains a controversial issue. Interobserver agreement in the reading of fetal heart rate tracings never exceeds 64% (6,7). Division of fetal heart rate tracings into segments of baseline, accelerations, and decelerations is a major problem, even for experienced obstetricians (8). Antepartum FHR testing has low sensitivity and a high rate of false positives. Results from EFM with regard to prediction of fetal outcome are comparable to fetal movement counting (9).

The rapid introduction and wide scale application of cardiotocography in obstetric practice was primarily based upon empirical evidence. Randomized trials followed decades later. After a period of overestimated appraisal, the technique is currently under attack. A committee of the Institute of Medicine of the National Academy of Sciences in the United States in 1989 even concluded that "Americans have adopted cardiotocography as standard practice, at considerable added expense to routine obstetrical care, despite the failure of scientific evidence to support its use" (10). Nevertheless, daily obstetric care relies substantially on the application of cardiotocography. Improvement of fetal surveillance became the primary goal of the European Community–sponsored concerted action project "New Methods for Perinatal Surveillance." One of the subprojects was defined to examine reasons for the low validity of cardiotocography (sensitivity 30–50%; specificity 90–92%) (11). Twenty-two well-known obstetricians from ten European Community countries were invited to participate in a study on classification and interpretation of cardiotocograms in relation to obstetric decision making.

Panel of Referees

The 21 obstetricians were brought into a classroom environment. Actual obstetric cases were presented to this panel of referees. The cases originated from a database of high-risk obstetric patient files collected within the European Community. The referees received extensive data on medical and obstetric history, course of pregnancy, the complete cardiotocographic recordings, and information from additional monitoring of maternal and fetal condition. The data were presented up to a certain point in time, when the referees had to read and interpret the cardiotocographic tracings, assess fetal condition, and decide upon obstetric management.

In total, 13 cases were submitted. Decision points included antepartum situations ($n = 3$) and intrapartum events during the first ($n = 5$) or second stage ($n = 5$) of labor. At each decision point the referees were asked to fill in a questionnaire and to segment and characterize the cardiotocographic tracing preceding the decision point. Classification of FHR phenomena was according to Hon (Table 1). In addition the referees were asked to assess subjectively the cardiotocographic tracing as normal, possibly abnormal, abnormal, or highly abnormal (terminal).

TABLE 1. *Classification scheme for fetal heart rhythm features*

Baseline variability	
increased	BI
normal	BN
reduced	BR
silent	BS
Acceleration	A
Deceleration	
early	DE
variable	DV
late	DL
other	DO
Undefined	U

The data derived from the segmented and classified cardiotocographic tracings were stored per referee in a MUMPS database, which was converted into so-called classification profiles for each type of fetal heart rate segment (12). The amplitude of a profile signal is equal to the number of referees classifying that particular characteristic of the fetal heart rate at each moment.

CLASSIFICATION AND INTERPRETATION OF CARDIOTOCOGRAPHIC TRACINGS

A summary of the referees' assessment of fetal condition compared with assessment of FHR tracings is presented in Table 2. A "normal" tracing was considered to be associated with a normal fetal condition in most instances. The same but opposite phenomenon was apparent for the traces assessed as "highly abnormal." However, unequivocal opinions appeared to be present in a majority of the cases, although the cases selected for presentation were not collected in a random fashion. In about two-thirds of the decision points, FHR traces were assessed as "possibly abnormal" or "abnormal." In these cases the interpretation of the traces was associated with an ambiguous estimation of fetal condition.

TABLE 2. *Assessment of fetal heart rate: cardiotocography (CTG) traces versus assessment of fetal condition*

	Fetal condition			
CTG	Good	Possibly endangered	Endangered	Severely endangered
Normal	53	6	—	—
Possibly abnormal	22	69	7	—
Abnormal	—	35	68	—
Highly abnormal	—	—	6	7

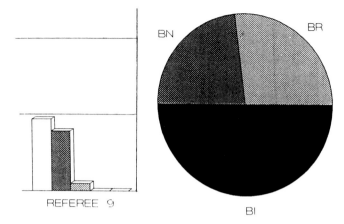

FIG. 1. Deceleration types and baseline variability by referee 9. The bars represent deceleration types from left to right: early, variable, late, other decelerations, and no classification. The pie chart represents distribution of baseline variability. BN, normal baseline variability; BI, variability increased; BR, variability reduced.

The major reason for the variation in assessment of fetal condition is a considerable difference in subjective assessment of the cardiotocographic tracings among the referees. Major differences were observed among the various referees in reading and describing exactly the same FHR traces. Examples are given in Figs. 1 and 2, representing the classification of deceleration types and baseline variability by two of

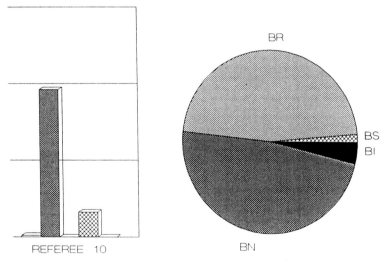

FIG. 2. Deceleration types and baseline variability by referee 10. The bars represent deceleration types from left to right: early, variable, late, other decelerations, and no classification. The pie chart represents distribution of baseline variability. BN, normal baseline variability; BI, variability increased; BR, variability reduced; BS, variability silent.

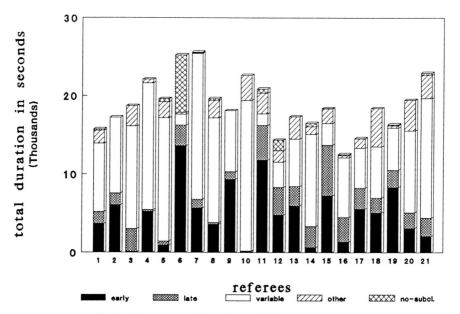

FIG. 3. Classification of baseline variability by the 21 referees.

the referees, both having looked at exactly the same traces. Although referee 9 considered about half the baseline segments to have increased variability, referee 10 recognized increased variability in only a small proportion of baseline segments. Whereas referee 9 classified FHR decelerations as either early or variable in nearly half the instances, referee 10 regarded decelerations as variable almost exclusively. This latter referee classified only a very few decelerations as early and none as late.

An overview of each referee's assessment of baseline variability and deceleration types is presented in Figs. 3 and 4. Obstetricians apparently differ greatly regarding their frame of reference.

FACTORS CAUSING DIFFICULTIES IN READING AND INTERPRETING FHR TRACES

A number of factors may explain the difficulties encountered in reading and interpreting FHR traces. One or more of the following factors may contribute:

1. The FHR pattern is too indirect a measure of fetal condition.
2. The FHR pattern primarily represents fetal central nervous system (CNS) functioning. Fetal circulatory and cardiac functioning is apparent only in cases of a deteriorating fetal condition.
3. Cardiotocography should be considered merely a screening method and should not be applied as a diagnostic tool.

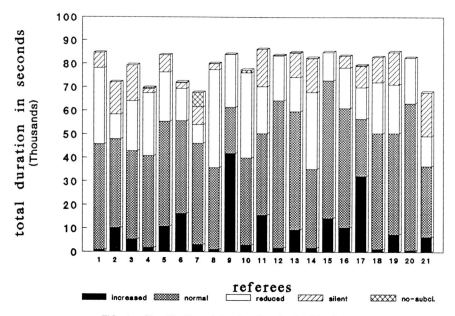

FIG. 4. Classification of decelerations by the 21 referees.

4. Visual analysis of FHR traces creates, among obstetricians, large differences in assessment of FHR features such as accelerations, decelerations, and variability. Exact criteria are not commonly accepted.
5. Even if criteria have been accepted they are very loosely applied. Visual analysis of FHR traces often lacks discipline.
6. Many factors involve the final FHR pattern (Table 3). The obstetrician reading a FHR tracing should be aware of the complexity of the end result of all these factors.

Interpretation of fetal heart rate patterns requires full knowledge of all clinical

TABLE 3. *Influences on fetal heart rate and variability*

Mother	Fetus
Drugs	Age
Fever, infection	Behavioral states
Hyperthyroidism	Circadian rhythms
Position	Congenital anomalies
Convulsions, shock	Cardiac innervation
	Brain damage
	Hypoxia

factors such as duration of pregnancy and maternal medication. The obstetrician should have in mind the concept of fetal behavioral states and should be able to conceptualize the actual situation with regard to fetal CNS and circulatory functioning.

IMPROVEMENT OF FHR MONITORING

Classification of FHR Patterns

First of all, adequate baseline recognition is essential. This requires a look at the full length of a tracing, lasting for a minimum of 30 min. "Jogging" of the fetus, hiccups (13), and maternal medication such as beta-mimetics can cause an increase in the baseline heart rate.

Visual analysis of full-length recording prevents variable decelerations from being classified incorrectly as early or late. The flow sheet published by Hon in 1968 (14) in his guidelines, *An Atlas of Fetal Heart Rate Patterns*, stresses the necessity first to observe whether "the FHR pattern reflects the waveform of uterine contraction." If this is not the case, decelerations are automatically classified as "variable decelerations." To quote Hon again: "The FHR pattern of variable deceleration is of prime importance in clinical obstetrics. It is the offending deceleration pattern in about 90 percent of the patients who have been clinically diagnosed as having fetal distress."

The Concept of Fetal Behavioral States

With improving resolution capacity of ultrasound equipment it became more and more attractive to study fetal behavioral states. Since respiration is not continuously present in fetal life and the existence of open or closed eyes is hardly recognizable in the fetus, other criteria for fetal behavioral states were required than are applied to the newborn infant (15). In 1982, Nijhuis and coworkers (16) proposed criteria for fetal behavioral states. Presence or absence of fetal eye and body movements and the heart rate pattern (HRP) were included in their criteria. Four fetal behavioral states were described, 1F to 4F, in analogy to the neonatal states 1 to 4. Their definitions of behavioral state are as follows:

State 1F: Eye and body movements absent, HRP A.
State 2F: Eye and (periodic) body movements present, HRP B.
State 3F: Eye movements present, body movements absent, HRP C.
State 4F: Eye and (continuous) body movements present, HRP D.

The fetal heart rate patterns A to D are defined as follows:

HPR A (state 1F): Stable heart rate with a narrow oscillation bandwidth.

HPR B (state 2F): Wider oscillation bandwidth than pattern A, with frequent accelerations in association with movements.

HPR C (state 3F): Stable heart rate with a wider oscillation bandwidth than pattern A and a more regular oscillation frequency than pattern B. There are no accelerations.

HPR D (state 4F): Unstable heart rate pattern, showing large and long-lasting accelerations, often fused into sustained tachycardia.

This behavioral-state concept has been widely accepted. Originally it was claimed that behavioral states could only be identified from 36 weeks of gestation onward. Before 36 weeks of gestation, however, coordination among the cycling patterns of heart rate variation, eye movements, and body movements is already present, suggesting a more or less gradual development of behavioral states (17,18). Fetal behavioral states are also recognizable during active labor (19). Within states, there is a close relationship between movements and heart rate phenomena (20–22). In the healthy fetus, the heart rate pattern is strongly influenced by type, duration, and timing of movements.

Automated Analysis of FHR

From the foregoing it is clear that uniform and disciplined classification of baseline and accelerations, decelerations, and variability appears virtually impossible in daily obstetric practice. It gives rise to a wide variety of opinions on the assessment of fetal condition and related obstetric management.

In recent years, stimulated especially by Professor Dawes in Oxford, successful attempts have been made to produce a system for automated analysis of FHR (23–25). This system has been commercialized and released by Oxford Sonicaid Medical Systems. Currently it is being tested in a randomized trial on conventional monitoring versus computerized FHR monitoring within the European Community concerted action project "New Methods for Perinatal Surveillance" (26). Automated analysis of FHR allows further investigations on the relationships between fetal (patho)physiologic variables (27,28).

CONCLUSIONS

Reading and interpreting FHR patterns requires knowledge about all factors that can influence sympathetic and parasympathetic regulation of fetal heart rhythm such as gestational age, maternal medication and type, and duration and timing of fetal movements. It is necessary to be thoroughly aware of the concept of fetal behavioral states. Further studies are required to understand fully the physiologic and pathophysiologic mechanisms at the basis of fetal heart rhythms. Future prospects include quantitative automated analysis of FHR patterns. Finally, it is necessary to integrate the conclusions on individual FHR patterns into a general concept in which clinical, biochemical, and biophysical data referring to fetal condition should be in harmony.

REFERENCES

1. Caldeyro-Barcia R, Mendez-Bauer C, Poseiro JJ, *et al*. Control of human fetal heart rate during labor. In: Cassels DE, ed. *The heart and circulation in the newborn and infant*. New York: Grune and Stratton, 1966;7.
2. Hon E, Quilligan EJ. Electronic evaluation of fetal heart rate. *Clin Obstet Gynecol* 1968;11:145–67.
3. Hammacher K. The diagnosis of fetal distress with an electronic fetal heart rate monitor. In: *Intrauterine dangers to the foetus*. Proceedings from a symposium in Prague. Amsterdam: Excerpta Medica, 1967;228.
4. Zuspan FP, Quilligan EJ, Iams JD, van Geijn HP. NICHD Consensus Development Task Force Report. Predictors of intrapartum fetal distress; the role of electronic fetal heart rate monitoring. *Am J Obstet Gynecol* 1979;135:287–91.
5. Low JA, Pancham SR, Worthington DN. Intrapartum fetal heart profiles with and without fetal asphyxia. *Am J Obstet Gynecol* 1977;127:729–37.
6. Van Geijn HP. Value and interpretation of fetal heart rate patterns. In: Clinch J, Matthews T, eds. *Perinatal medicine*. Lancaster: MTP Press, 1985;71.
7. Trimbos JB, Keirse MJNC. Observer variability in assessment of antepartum cardiotocograms. *Br J Obstet Gynaecol* 1978;85:900–6.
8. Van Geijn HP, Donker DK, Derom R, Duisterhout JS, Copray FJA. Interventions based upon cardiotocographic recordings. In: Di Renzo G, Cosmi E, eds. *Proceedings XI European Congress of Perinatal Medicine*. Chur: Harwood Academic Publishers, 1989;446–53.
9. Thacker SB, Berkelman RL. Assessing the diagnostic accuracy and efficacy of selected antepartum fetal surveillance techniques. *Obstet Gynecol Survey* 1986;41:121–41.
10. Rostow VP, Osterweis M, Bulger RJ. Medical professional liability and the delivery of obstetrical care. *N Engl J Med* 1989;321:1057–60.
11. Jongsma HW, Eskes TKAB. Validity of electronic fetal monitoring: a comparative study in seven university hospitals. In: Di Renzo G, Cosmi E, eds. *Proceedings XI European Congress of Perinatal Medicine*. Chur: Harwood Academic Publishers, 1989;439–45.
12. Donker DK, van Geijn HP, Jongsma HW, Duisterhout JS, de Moel EJPM. Processing and presentation of visually coded and interpreted fetal heart rate patterns. In: Salomon R, Blum J, Jorgensen M, eds. *MEDINFO 86*, part 2. Amsterdam: Elsevier Science Publishers, 1986;693–5.
13. Van Woerden EE, van Geijn HP, Caron FJM, Swartjes JM, Arts NFTh. Fetal hiccups; characteristics and relation to fetal heart rate. *Eur J Obstet Gynecol Reprod Biol* 1989;30:209–16.
14. Hon EH. *An atlas of fetal heart rate patterns*. New Haven: Harty Press Inc, 1968.
15. Van Geijn HP, Jongsma HW, De Haan J, Eskes TKAB, Prechtl HFR. Heart rate as an indicator of the behavioral state; studies in the newborn and prospects for fetal heart rate monitoring. *Am J Obstet Gynecol* 1980;136:1061–6.
16. Nijhuis JG, Prechtl HFR, Martin Jr CB, Bots RSGM. Are there behavioural states in the human fetus? *Early Hum Devel* 1982;6:177–95.
17. Visser GHA, Poelmann-Weesjes G, Cohen TMN, Bekedam DJ. Fetal behaviour at 30–32 weeks of gestation. *Pediatr Res* 1987;22:655–8.
18. Swartjes JM, van Geijn HP, Mantel R, van Woerden EE, Schoemaker HC. Coincidence of behavioral state parameters in the human fetus at three gestational ages. *Early Hum Devel* 1990;23:75–83.
19. Griffin RL, Caron FJM, van Geijn HP. Behavioural states in the human fetus during labor. *Am J Obstet Gynecol* 1985;152:828–33.
20. Van Woerden EE, van Geijn HP, Swartjes JM, Caron FJM, Brons JTJ, Arts NFTh. Fetal heart rhythms during behavioural state 1F. *Eur J Obstet Gynecol Reprod Biol* 1988;28:29–38.
21. Van Woerden EE, van Geijn HP, Caron FJM, Swartjes JM, Mantel R. Automated assignment of behavioural states in the human near term fetus. *Early Hum Devel* 1989;19:137–46.
22. Van Woerden EE, van Geijn HP, Caron FJM, Mantel R. Spectral analysis of fetal heart rhythm in relation to fetal regular mouthing. *Int J Biomed Comput* 1990;25:253–60.
23. Dawes GS, Redman CGW, Smith JH. Improvements in the registration and analysis of fetal heart rate records at the bedside. *Br J Obstet Gynaecol* 1985;92:317–25.
24. Dawes GS, Moulden M, Redman CWG. Criteria for the design of fetal heart rate analysis systems. *Int J Biomed Comput* 1990;25:287–94.
25. Dawes GS, Moulden M, Redman CWG. The advantages of computerized fetal heart rate analysis. *J Perinatal Med* 1991;19(1/2):39–45.

26. Van Geijn HP, Jongsma HW, Derom R, Eskes TKAB, eds. Personal computer based analysis of fetal heart rate. *Int J Biomed Comput* 1990;25:235–7.
27. Mantel R, van Geijn HP, Caron FJM, Swartjes JM, van Woerden EE, Jongsma HW. Computer analysis of antepartum fetal heart rate: 1. Baseline determination. *Int J Biomed Comput* 1990;25:261–72.
28. Mantel R, van Geijn HP, Caron FJM, Swartjes JM, van Woerden EE, Jongsma HW. Computer analysis of antepartum fetal heart rate: 2. Detection of accelerations and decelerations. *Int J Biomed Comput* 1990;25:273–86.

DISCUSSION

Dr. Dawes: How accurate are these new methods? How does the phono compare with the direct ECG, for example.

Dr. Van Geijn: We are examining this at the moment in a collaborative investigation between our department of medical physics and the obstetric department, using the phono transducer primarily to detect respiratory movements in the fetus. When we compare ultrasound observations with the phono data it is clear that in many instances breathing movements can be readily detected with the phono system. It must therefore be able to detect fetal body movements. We are currently testing how the phono system handles fetal heart rate, uterine contractions, and fetal body movements.

Dr. Hobel: Fetal assessment is especially important when there is meconium in the amniotic fluid. In the cases you presented to your panel, did any of them have meconium? How did the physicians handle this situation?

Dr. Van Geijn: We gave the panel all the information available, so if there was meconium we informed them. The primary aim was to see how they handled the heart rate patterns and I do not know how they dealt with the meconium problem as an individual variable. However, I fully agree with you that meconium is a clinical feature that should be considered very carefully. The recent study by Rossi, *et al.* (1) again demonstrated the strong relationship between fresh meconium and certain heart rate patterns, in particular the absence of accelerations, a slight increase in baseline heart rate, and the association with postmaturity.

Dr. Guesry: I am struck by the fact that, since your study was retrospective, you knew the actual outcome. You knew what should have been a good answer to the cardiotocographic and other findings. Have you compared the panel's answer to the ideal answer? Was the response of the clinicians in charge of these particular cases better than average? Maybe the actual decision was better than it could have been from a panel of people who were divorced from the clinical reality.

Dr. Van Geijn: You are correct that the panel did not know about the outcome. Having studied the cases I am convinced that the clinicians in charge of the cases did no better than the panel would have done. All the panel members agreed that the cases were presented in an appropriate way and close to the real clinical situation. It was after all not much different from the usual day-to-day situation when a resident or colleague comes with a case and presents you, as a staff member, with the clinical data.

What the study proved was that even obstetricians who are experts in fetal heart monitoring and surveillance have the same difficulties as average clinicians in a district hospital. Many other studies over the past 5 or 10 years have shown the same results. What we were especially interested in was why cardiotocography does not fulfill clinical expectations. I suspect there are many reasons for this. One is that heart rate is too indirect a parameter, relating primarily to the function of the central nervous system and having little bearing on cardiac metabolic function. Only when the fetal condition deteriorates does it reflect cardiac function to some extent. Second, we are badly educated on the meaning and definition of heart rate patterns. There are at least 20 definitions and nobody sticks to any of them. Obstetricians are very undisciplined in looking at heart rate patterns. Nobody really does it in the way I presented: reading, description, interpretation. And I think that many obstetricians are not aware of the wide variation in normal fetal heart rate patterns, many of which are erroneously considered abnormal.

Dr. Jouppila: Our problem with cardiotocography (CTG) is that we have so many false-positive results. Using pH determinations we can markedly decrease the number of false-positive CTG interpretations, and I believe these should be done on a regular basis, particularly in university departments where there are many young doctors in training.

Dr. Van Geijn: In the study by Jongsma and Eskes (2) it was shown that the sensitivity of CTG was about 30%. When fetal blood sampling was used in addition, the sensitivity increased to nearly 50%. I agree with you. We should encourage fetal blood sampling in labor.

Dr. Hope: I think the results of your study were determined by your selection of cases rather than by the accuracy of the technique.

Dr. Van Geijn: I agree in general that selection can be an important factor, but I am strongly convinced that the cases used were typical of those that occur daily in normal clinical practice.

Dr. Dawes: A recent study by John Patrick and his colleagues in London, Ontario, is relevant. John Patrick died earlier this year and I don't know when the studies will be published. They were covering 100 records circulated on three occasions, mixed-up, to the same five observers, all of whom were expert in CTG analysis. The research team used the kappa statistic to assess inter- and intraobserver reliability. They came to the same general conclusion as Prof. van Geijn, that evaluation of heart rate variability was statistically not different from random, and assessment of baseline heart rate was hardly any better. When there was more than one deceleration on a record, there was a 40% variation in interpretation between individuals or by the same individual a month or two later. These are astonishing inconsistencies in visual interpretation of CTG records.

REFERENCES

1. Rossi EM, Philipson EH, Williams TG, Kalhan SC. Meconium aspiration syndrome: intrapartum and neonatal attributes. *Am J Obstet Gynecol* 1989;161:1106–10.
2. Jongsma HW, Eskes TKAB. Validity of electronic fetal monitoring: a comparative study in seven university hospitals. In: Di Renzo G, Cosmi E, eds. *Proceedings XI European Congress of Perinatal Medicine*. Chur: Harwood Academic Publishers, 1989;439–45.

Perinatology, edited by Erich Saling,
Nestlé Nutrition Workshop Series, Vol. 26,
Nestec, Ltd., Vevey/Raven Press, Ltd.,
New York © 1992.

Computerised Evaluation of the Fetal Heart Rate Trace

Geoffrey S. Dawes

*Nuffield Department of Obstetrics and Gynaecology, University of Oxford,
John Radcliffe Hospital, Oxford OX3 9DU, United Kingdom*

Dr. Redman and I joined forces to undertake a computerised evaluation of antenatal fetal heart rate (FHR) traces (with tocodynamometer and fetal movement counts) in 1978. He, like many others, had found it impossible to fit a baseline to the FHR satisfactorily by eye or by using a pencil and ruler. It was a comparatively straightforward matter to design a computer programme to fit the FHR baseline in the first thousand records (1). The principles have remained the same, but with increased experience small adaptations have been made to allow for the astonishing variety of records, especially in deteriorating fetuses.

By 1986 we had a relatively sophisticated analysis program running on-line using a fast modern personal computer (Apricot Xen), accessed to an HP8040 fetal monitor, and were able to draw on the experience gained and the record archive accumulated over the previous 5 years. Oxford Sonicaid adapted the software (rewriting it in C, in place of Pascal) and made it available commercially in February 1989. In the meantime we had also collected the experience of many friends, notably Gerry Visser in Groningen, John Patrick in London, Ontario, and GianPaulo Mandruzzato in Trieste, as well as a small clinical trial undertaken by Tim Wheeler in Southampton and Mike Lobb in Luton and Dunstable. So we now have access to an archive of some 15,000 records from Oxford and another 14,000 from Trieste and the clinical trial in England.

The advantages of a computerised analysis are several. First the program is interactive, so that the midwife or other operator is advised at once of excessive signal loss by audible and visual signals. This halved signal loss in the clinical trial in Southampton. In addition the data are scrutinised by error algorithms, which reject abrupt deviations upward or downward from the baseline fetal heart rate with an equally abrupt return, attributed to the limitations of the fetal monitors (2). The use of a computer has many other advantages. It removes the relatively large intra- and interobserver variation and it optimises the use of time by advising the midwife to stop recording as soon as the computer has identified a feature that shows that the FHR trace is normal. The average time of recording is about 15 min, varying between 10 min for a very normal trace and 60 min for a highly abnormal trace. In

Southampton if the midwives had followed the recommendation of the computer they would have saved themselves and the patients 800 hours of recording time in the year. There is a further notable benefit to the use of computerised analysis, in that it becomes easy for a junior doctor to give a clear numerical description of a puzzling FHR record to his supervisor over the telephone at night. Thus it improves communication.

DIAGNOSTIC DISCRIMINATION USING COMPUTERISED RECORDS

Antenatal Traces

I particularly want to draw attention to the improvement in diagnostic discrimination that has resulted from analysis of the antenatal archive. Some years ago Visser and Huisjes (3) and Visser et al. (4) gave an important description of preterminal and terminal FHR traces. We can now attribute numerical values to these. For example if FHR variation is reduced from the normal value of about 45 ms (mean range of *long-term* variation in pulse interval) to 20 ms in association with growth retardation or/and pre-eclamptic toxaemia, then the fetus will have developed chronic hypoxaemia but will not yet be acidaemic (5,6). Some such fetuses continue to deteriorate and a few may develop not only a further decrease in FHR variation but superimposed on that a sinusoidal variation of small amplitude. The effect of this sinusoidal pattern can be eliminated by using an index of short-term variation ($\frac{1}{16}$ min epoch-to-epoch variation) which is a reliable guide to the onset of acidaemia, as it falls below 2.5 ms (from a normal value in excess of 7 ms). The presence of this progressive decrease in FHR variation is a more reliable index of impending death from acidaemia than is the presence of repeated decelerations. The presence of decelerations may be a warning sign but their incidence, duration, amplitude, and area are not correlated with the decline in short-term variation in FHR. We therefore conclude that as a *single measure of abnormality* short-term FHR variation is to be preferred. In eight instances since 1984 impending fetal death was diagnosed by a fall in short-term FHR variation well below 2.5 ms. A decision was taken not to deliver these fetuses by Caesarean section because of immaturity and severe growth retardation. All died within 24 hours.

However, *as a measure of normality* the presence of episodes of high long-term FHR variation corresponding to active sleep are preferred, because this measure takes account of prolonged accelerations lasting more than a minute. It is more reliable than counting accelerations, as in the non-stress test (7), since many younger fetuses, as well as a few older than 34 weeks, have few or no accelerations of the amplitude and duration normally stipulated in the course of even an hour's recording. This accounts for the high false-positive feature of non-stress tests, estimated visually.

In summary then, computerised FHR analysis antenatally provides a better identification of normal FHR traces and, using a measure of short-term FHR variation, a good measure of abnormal traces. Wider experience is still required to establish the limits of this measurement; the last word is not yet said on this subject.

Labour Traces

If computerised FHR analysis produces a new interpretation antenatally, can it be equally effective when applied to labour traces? Five years ago Dr Redman and I started to collect FHR records in labour, through Prof. Colin Mantell who took a period of sabbatical leave in Oxford and through Laura Pello who accumulated 500 good-quality records over a couple of years, with blood gas analyses available on delivery in 394. Since that time Dr Orla Sheil has accumulated records of nearly 30 traces from fetuses diagnosed as asphyxiated at birth and almost 2,000 controls. The analysis of these data, with the help of Dr Sylvia Rosevear, has proved complex and time-consuming. However, there are some principles which have emerged.

Spencer and Johnson reported in 1986 (8) that, on visual analysis, episodic rest/ activity cycles persisted in labour throughout the first stage and, as one of their figures showed, into the second stage. The interobserver variation was recorded as 11% but not defined; we assume that this reflected disagreement about the presence or absence of episodic cycling. Our analysis of 137 records, in which at least 4 h of good-quality recording was available before the start of the second stage, showed that the amplitude and duration of both low and high FHR variation, characteristic of rest/activity cycles, corresponded closely with those seen before the onset of labour. The importance of this observation requires further consideration. The amplitude of FHR variation *in episodes of low variation*, characteristic of quiet sleep antenatally or in labour, approximates to that observed *continuously* in fetuses liable to impending death *in utero* (preterminal to terminal according to Visser and Huisjes's classification). When Hon, Beard, Kubli, and others described attenuation of FHR variation (a very flat trace, less than 5 bpm variation) as a sinister sign they were unaware of the fact that there was such episodic low variation antenatally; it was first described in the human in 1978, though it had already been observed in fetal lambs (9). Therefore we must review those traces in which it has been alleged that a flat feature, pathognomonic of impending acidaemia, is present and ask whether this is not simply an episode of normal FHR variation, or whether the fetus was already compromised before the onset of labour. The material already presented in the obstetric journals is not adequate to answer this question.

Our own measurements in labour of either FHR or of FHR variation so far show no statistical correlation with outcome as measured by arterial blood gas values at delivery or by Apgar score or by identification of those fetuses subsequently admitted to the special care baby unit with a diagnosis of "asphyxia at birth". Neither alone, nor in combination with other FHR variables, do they significantly improve discrimination. We are led to question the guidelines as to the normal distribution of FHR and FHR variation, accepted for the last 100 years and more as a result first of auscultation and latterly by electronic fetal monitoring. Our own archive of labour material is still small. The basal FHR already exceeds the limits of 120–160 bpm early in the first stage; with the progress of labour the spread is further increased at either end (below 120 and above 160 bpm), with normal outcome. FHR variation normally varies widely and episodically in labour. Had this material been available when the FIGO Committee issued its most recent assessment of the position (10), attention would have been drawn to it. Adequate computer data bases must now be prepared from which to derive the truth. There is still a real possibility that FHR analysis may help to discriminate between acidaemic or damaged fetuses in labour and those with a normal outcome, but it must be done objectively with a computer.

SUMMARY

A brief description is given of some of the advantages of the use of computerised fetal heart rate (FHR) analysis antenatally interactive and on-line. These include: (a) consistent objective analysis, independent of observer variation based on an archive of thousands of records; (b) greater accuracy, with reduced signal loss and automatic elimination of errors arising from the limitations of current fetal monitors; (c) better use of time, varying from 10 min (and by increments of 2 min thereafter according to fetal rest-activity cycles) up to 60 min for a highly abnormal record, *with an average of 15 min*; (d) automatic recall of previous records on the same patient, to provide material for a synoptic review over periods up to 4 weeks; (e) improved identification of FHR traces with normal outcome, by measurement of episodes of high FHR variation associated with activity cycles; and (f) improved analysis of abnormal FHR traces by measurement of short-term variation, and hence identification of preterminal and terminal traces, characteristic of hypoxaemia, alone or combined with acidaemia. This is based on blood gas measurements on delivery or on death *in utero*.

A short account is given of preliminary observations on records made during labour. These show the persistence of rest-activity cycles, in which the amplitude of variation (during "rest cycles") falls to a value no different from that observed in terminal FHR traces antenatally. This casts doubt on the allegation that short episodes (up to 1 h in length) of low FHR variation are of sinister significance diagnostically. Neither FHR nor FHR variation showed a statistically significant relationship with outcome measured by arterial blood gas values on delivery, Apgar score, or admission to special care for "birth asphyxia". The guidelines need revision by the use of well-authenticated computerised data bases.

REFERENCES

1. Dawes GS, Houghton R, Redman CWG. Baseline in human fetal heart rate records. *Br J Obstet Gynaecol* 1982;89:270–5.
2. Dawes GS, Moulden M, Redman CWG. Limitations of antenatal fetal heart rate monitors. *Am J Obstet Gynecol* 1990;162:170–3.

3. Visser GHA, Huisjes HJ. Diagnostic value of the unstressed antepartum CTG. *Br J Obstet Gynaecol* 1977;84:321–6.
4. Visser GHA, Huisjes HJ, Redman CWG, Turnbull AC. Non-stressed antepartum heart-rate monitoring implications of decelerations after spontaneous contractions. *Am J Obstet Gynecol* 1980;138:429–35.
5. Henson G, Dawes GS, Redman CWG. Antenatal fetal heart rate variability in relation to fetal acid-base status at caesarean section. *Br J Obstet Gynaecol* 1983;90:516–21.
6. Smith JH, Anand KJS, Cotes PM, *et al.* Antenatal fetal heart rate variation in relation to the respiratory and metabolic status of the compromised human fetus. *Br J Obstet Gynaecol* 1988;95:980–9.
7. Dawes GS, Houghton R, Redman CWG, Visser GHA. Pattern of the normal human fetal heart rate. *Br J Obstet Gynaecol* 1982;89:276–84.
8. Spencer JAD, Johnson P. Fetal heart rate variability changes and fetal behavioural cycles during labour. *Br J Obstet Gynaecol* 1986;93:314–21.
9. Dalton KJ, Dawes GS, Patrick JE. Diurnal, respiratory and other rhythms of the fetal heart rate in lambs. *Am J Obstet Gynecol* 1977;127:414–24.
10. Rooth G, Huch H, Huch R. Guidelines for the use of fetal monitoring. *Int J Gynecol Obstet* 1987;25:159–67.

DISCUSSION

Dr. Saling: I am confused about the results you have observed so often: hypoxaemic features but lack of acidaemia. Which cases show this combination and what is the borderline between normality and acidosis or acidaemia?

Dr. Dawes: Many experiments performed in various parts of the world have shown a characteristic train of events when fetal lambs have been exposed to hypoxia for periods of up to a week or more. Within the first few minutes the heart rate falls, the blood pressure rises, and fetal limb and breathing movements cease. There is not uncommonly a mild degree of acidaemia during the first 6 h. But by 12 or 24 h the acidaemia has gone, heart rate and heart rate variation return to normal values, breathing movements are regained, and limb movements are also restored within 24 h. Plasma erythropoietin has risen by this time, but there is no effect yet on haemoglobin. We have no satisfactory explanation for this remarkable phenomenon, i.e., that sheep fetuses adapt to chronic hypoxaemia within 24 h. In human fetuses with growth retardation, long-term heart rate variation is reduced to 20 ms (short-term variation about 3.5 ms). When such fetuses are delivered by caesarean section in the absence of labour, the PO_2 is reduced from a normal value of about 13 mm Hg to about 6 mm Hg, a highly significant difference. There is no evidence of metabolic acidaemia in this situation but erythropoietin concentration is increased fourfold. So human fetuses attempt the same kind of adaptation as the sheep fetus *in utero*, and these results have been confirmed by cordocentesis (1).

I feel hesitant about speculating on the mechanism by which fetal heart rate variation is reduced. Smith (2) took a set of human infants delivered by caesarean section in the absence of labour, with a flat fetal heart rate trace and chronic hypoxia. Average PO_2 was about 6 mm Hg. These infants were not acidaemic, nor did they develop respiratory distress in the next 24 h. He followed the change in fetal heart rate variability after delivery, when the PO_2 rose toward the normal infant value of 60–80 mm Hg. There was no immediate change in heart rate variation. It took 24 h for the variation to reach normal values. Thus the reduced variability is unlikely to be directly due to the hypoxaemia.

Dr. Saling: What about the PCO_2?

Dr. Dawes: Arterial PCO_2 in growth retarded fetuses with a flat heart rate trace is commonly a little raised; instead of being in the low 40s (mm Hg) it is in the low 50s, and there is a slight respiratory acidaemia. This is unlikely to explain the low heart rate variability; in sheep or rhesus monkeys hypercapnia causes *increased* heart rate variability.

Dr. Hope: I am interested that an animal fetus that has been chronically hypoxic may compensate its acidosis. This fits in with two sets of clinical observations. One is the work of Ann Johnson and colleagues from Oxford (3) which showed a particularly poor outcome in infants with very low Apgar scores and normal cord artery pH—an unexpected finding and therefore more likely to be true. The other is our own anecdotal observation that some infants delivered because of a very abnormal CTG, where, in spite of severe asphyxia and subsequent devastating neonatal encephalopathy, there were nevertheless reasonable cord blood pH values. It does appear that some fetuses can be in serious trouble but be born with a normal blood pH. I therefore wonder whether pH at delivery is a suitable gold standard by which to assess the value of other tests of fetal condition.

Dr. Dawes: I am aware of your interesting observations. We are at present in the process of analysing a large data set of 2,000 normal deliveries and 30 babies born with an Apgar score of 3 or less. We shall examine this series to see whether or not low Apgar scores are associated with metabolic acidaemia.

Dr. Marini: What is your view about the Frank-Starling law in the fetal heart.

Dr. Dawes: The facts are well established. Twenty-five years ago Job Faber showed that Starling's law operated in the heart of the embryonic mouse at septation. In late gestation, Rudolph and others have shown that there is a large increase in cardiac contractility at birth. In the fetus, cardiac output rises as atrial distension is increased up to a certain maximum, but this maximum is low and the subsequent plateau is flat. As soon as the fetus is delivered, peak cardiac output increases and contractility rises twofold or more after birth. The most reasonable explanation for this is that the fetal chest is full of fluid; when the atrium contracts and pushes blood into the ventricle it has to displace lung liquid, and clearly this can limit cardiac output. Ventilation of the lungs, even with a gas mixture that causes no change in fetal oxygen or CO_2, enables the fetal heart to increase its contractility. This suggests a purely mechanical effect.

Dr. Hobel: You showed some data to indicate time course in observations of heart rate variability. Have you tried to classify this so that guidelines will be available for predicting the probability of some level of morbidity?

Dr. Dawes: I showed the data up to 1987. We have three more years' experience since then. About one-third of the 78 patients illustrated appeared to deteriorate rapidly. Often the first sign was a reduction in the fetal movement pattern, as indicated by the mother. In the remainder there was a reduction in fetal heart rate variability. At the other extreme there were cases where reduced heart rate variability continued for a month, with gradual deterioration. The synoptic display really is a help in this situation. In the future we must discover whether the decision to extend pregnancy from, say, 28 weeks to 30 weeks or from 29 weeks to 32 weeks, in the presence of chronic hypoxia, is causing damage. Prospective trials will have to be arranged. The current European multicentre trial will only tell us whether the computer system is useful in diagnosis in the short term. Longer term studies are important and we should start thinking ahead as to how these can be arranged.

Dr. Elser: I have a question concerning maternal conditions during antepartum cardioto-cography. Is there a difference depending on whether the mother is lying on the bed or moving about?

Dr. Dawes: We standardise the mother's position in a semirecumbent comfortable posture. We know there is a large diurnal variation in fetal heart rate and heart rate variability, the main change occurring in the early evening, so we make measurements during normal working hours (9 AM to 4 PM).

REFERENCES

1. Visser GHA, Sadovsky G, Nicolaides KH. Antepartum heart rate patterns in small for gestational age third trimester fetuses: correlations with blood gases obtained at cordocentesis. *Am J Obstet Gynecol* 1990;182:698–703.
2. Smith JH. *Low human fetal heart rate variation*. MD Thesis, University of Cambridge, 1989.
3. Dennis J, Johnson A, Mutch L, Yudkin P, Johnson P. Acid-base status at birth and neurodevelopmental outcome at four and one-half years. *Am J Obstet Gynecol* 1989;161:213–20.

Perinatology, edited by Erich Saling,
Nestlé Nutrition Workshop Series, Vol. 26,
Nestec, Ltd., Vevey/Raven Press, Ltd.,
New York © 1992.

Transabdominal Laserspectroscopy in Human Fetus During Labor

Stephan Schmidt, S. Gorissen, W. Decleer, H. Eilers,
and D. Krebs

*Department of Gynecology and Obstetrics, University of Bonn,
Sigmund Freud Strasse 25, 5300 Bonn, Germany*

The routinely used cardiotocography (CTG) has been criticized for the effect of leading to an unacceptably high number of cesarean sections (1,2). Information on biochemical variables leads to better identification of fetal distress (3–5).

The newly available laserspectroscopy provides information about biochemical variables in a continuous and noninvasive way, and thus might prove to be an adequate technique for fetal surveillance (6–10). In this chapter we report our first experiences with the transabdominal application of laser systems and their evaluation during simultaneous recording of CTG and transcutaneous PO_2 measurements in the fetus during labor. The aim of this analysis is to evaluate the reliability of laserspectroscopy in identifying critical changes of oxygenation.

METHOD

The radiometer prototype that was used comprises a Hewlett Packard personal computer interconnected with a near-infrared data collection unit (NIRDCU). The NIRDCU includes a transmitter board with four laser diodes with wavelengths of 775 nm, 805 nm, 845 nm, and 904 nm, as well as a microcomputer board with power supply. There is in addition a receiver module with an optical receiver, an amplifier, and a converter. The system is constructed in accordance with the research published by Rea and coworkers (9). Light from the laser diodes is conduced by means of optical fiber bundles to a prism located in the sensor. The reflected light is collected in a sensor and registered in the NIRDCU by means of photodiodes. Changes of the optical density in relation to the time are displayed on the monitor, while data are also stored for graphical processing.

The laser sensor incorporates two optical prisms. One provides divergent radiation and the other detects the reflected laser light. The sensor was applied to the abdominal wall directly over the fetal head (Fig. 1). The exact position of the fetal head was localized by means of ultrasound examinations.

87

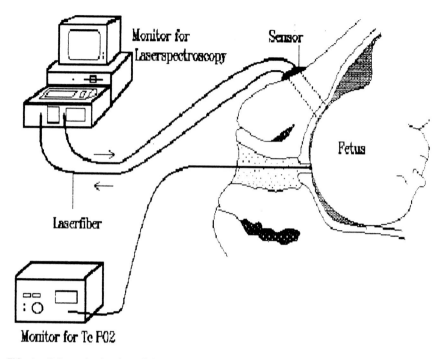

FIG. 1. Schematic drawing of the monitoring system for laserspectroscopy in the fetus during labor (Radiometer prototype). (i) Conduction of near-infrared laser light (NIR) from the laserdiodes to the patient; (ii) Conduction of reflected laser light from the sensor to the collection unit; (iii) Near-infrared collection unit (NIRDCU); (iv) Data processing and graphics.

Fetal blood samples were collected during labor by means of the Saling technique (11). Blood samples were analyzed in a Corning blood gas analyzer (Corning 178 pH). Transcutaneous PO_2 measurements were performed with the Radiometer TCM 3 Monitor. Details of the application of the electrode are reported elsewhere (4). Data collected simultaneously by all three methods were compared, and linear correlation coefficients were calculated. The measurements were performed in six primiparous women and four women in their second pregnancy. Combined monitoring with transcutaneous PO_2 measurements and laserspectroscopy over 480 min were analyzed. The sample frequency of values was generally 10 min. In addition, in cases with indications of fetal distress the preceeding10-min section of the fetal blood sample was analyzed with a sample frequency of 1 min.

RESULTS

Using transabdominal laserspectroscopy it was possible to trace changes in absorbances at four different wavelengths and to calculate relative changes of HbO_2, desaturated hemoglobin, total hemoglobin, and cytochrome aa_3. The changes in these

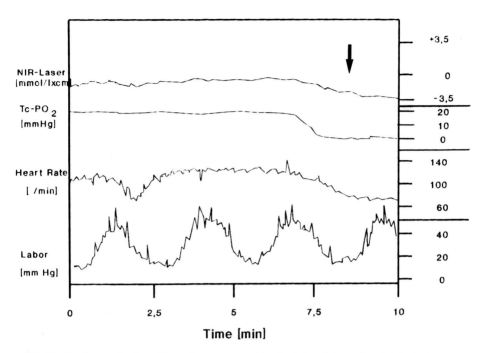

FIG. 2. Continuous tracing of laser signals representing the intracellular redox state (cytochrome aa_3), transcutaneous measured PO_2, fetal heart rate, and labor during an episode of fetal distress. The decrease of PO_2 indicated by the tracings is verified by fetal blood sampling (FBA). The fetal PO_2 was 8 mm Hg. The baby was born by forceps delivery. It was in a vigorous status (Apgar 7, 9, 10). The acidosis in the fetal blood was verified in a postpartum blood sample from the umbilical cord.

four biochemical variables, and in the CTG and the transcutaneous measurements of partial pressure of oxygen are shown graphically in Fig. 2.

In cases without fetal distress we observed stable values with only minor fluctuations related to changes of intrauterine pressure. On the other hand in cases where there was an intrauterine complication the deterioration of oxygenation was detected from a decrease in HbO_2 and cytochrome aa_3 values as well as from falling tc-PO_2 and PO_2 values in the fetal blood.

Figure 2 shows how the laserspectroscopic tracings of the different biochemical variables change during the development of an intrauterine disturbance.

As we can see in Fig. 3 there is a statistically significant linear correlation between the oxygenated hemoglobin calculated by means of laserspectroscopy and the partial pressure of oxygen measured transcutaneously, with a correlation coefficient $r = 0.90$. Additionally we found a linear correlation, with a correlation coefficient $r = 0.87$, between the transcutaneous PO_2 and the cytochrome aa_3 measured by the laserspectrometer (Fig. 4). The values of the transcutaneous PO_2 measurements were verified by comparing them with directly determined fetal blood values. Here the correlation coefficient was $r = 0.97$.

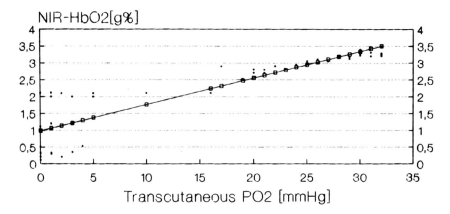

FIG. 3. Correlation of tc-PO$_2$ and NIR-HbO$_2$ measured by laserspectroscopy. Correlation coefficient r = 0.90; n = 57. •, NIR-HbO$_2$(g%); —⊟—, correlation of HbO$_2$/tc-PO$_2$. NIR-HbO$_2$ = 0.979 + 0.079 × tc-PO$_2$.

DISCUSSION

New techniques of fetal surveillance are of special interest, since CTG too often implicates fetal distress and thus leads to action by obstetricians in cases where the fetus is not really in danger (2,5). The additional techniques aimed at improving fetal monitoring have a number of shortcomings (12,13). The routine use of fetal blood sampling is supposed to be too cumbersome (11), and problems with tissue pH measurements and transcutaneous systems have up to now inhibited the routine use of these techniques. All these procedures are invasive in the sense that rupture of the

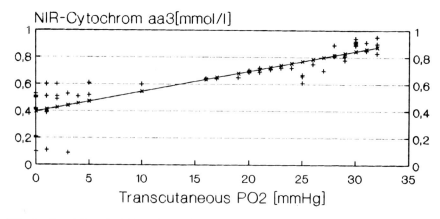

FIG. 4. Correlation of tc-PO$_2$ and the NIR-cytochrome aa$_3$ measured by laserspectroscopy. Correlation coefficient r = 0.87; n = 57. +, NIR-cytochrome aa$_3$; —✳—, correlation of cytochrome to tc-PO$_2$. NIR-cytochrome = 0.397 + 0.015 × tc-PO$_2$.

membranes and some penetration of the skin is essential (12,14–17). The transabdominal application of laser sensors was performed during a clinical trial aimed at evaluating this technique as an additional tool for fetal surveillance.

A number of objections against the general use of the different systems for biochemical fetal monitoring have been listed in the past. Transcutaneous monitors are supposed to be too complicated for routine use in the labor ward. Inconvenient application procedures including shaving of the fetal scalp have been proposed. Traumatization of the measuring site by the tissue pH electrode has prohibited the more widespread use of this technique. The use of transabdominal laserspectroscopy is a potential solution to these problems as it provides a continuous and noninvasive form of fetal monitoring, though the first laserspectroscopy ever performed was achieved after transvaginal application of the sensors directly on the fetal head (10).

During the clinical trial reported here the transabdominal application of the laserspectrometer sensor resulted in all ten cases in achievement of an optical signal sufficient to allow calculation of HbO_2, reduced hemoglobin, relative change of blood volume, and cytochrome aa_3. The reliability of laserspectroscopy was verified by comparison with results from intermittently collected fetal blood samples as well as with the continuous tracings of transcutaneous blood gas measurements (tc-PO_2). There was good correlation between simultaneously collected data from transcutaneous measurements and fetal blood samples when no hypoxia occurred. On the other hand tc-PO_2 values tended to underestimate PO_2 values in the range of 15–25 mm Hg. This might be explained by the influence of variable perfusion and edema of the skin on the transcutaneous measurements (15).

The detection of the laserspectroscopy signals provides a possibility of resolving suspect prepathological and pathological heart rate patterns that might otherwise result in the need for operative delivery. In this way a reduction in the number of cesarean sections might be achieved. Surprisingly, artifacts due to fetal and maternal movements had only a minor effect on laserspectroscopic tracings.

When any new technique is applied the occurrence of side effects should be reported. Laser pulses with a maximum length of 200 ns and a repetition frequency of 500 Hz result in a low optical output power of less than 4 mW. Additionally, according to the Planck-Einstein relation, the photon energy in the near-infrared range is supposed to be low. In conclusion we consider laserspectroscopy to be safe. We hope that the price of laserspectroscopy, as well as the relatively easy technique, will lead to the widespread use of such optical sensors in the future.

REFERENCES

1. Banta HD, Thacker S. Assessing the costs and benefits of electronic fetal monitoring. *Obstet Gynecol Surv* 1979;34:627.
2. Sykes GS, Molloy PM, Johnson P, Stirrat GM, Turnbull AC. Fetal distress and the condition of newborn infants. *Br Med J* 1983;287:943.
3. Saling E. Fetal scalp blood analysis. *J Perinat Med* 1981;9:165.
4. Schmidt S. Methodology and clinical value of transcutaneous blood gas measurements in the fetus. *J Perinat Med* 1988;16:95–107.

5. van den Berg P, Schmidt S, Gesche J, Saling E. Fetal distress and the condition of the newborn using cardiotocography and the fetal blood analysis during labour. *Br J Obstet Gynaecol* 1987;94:72.
6. Brazy JE, Lewis DV, Mitnick MH, Jöbsis van der Vliet FF. Noninvasive monitoring of cerebral oxygenation in preterm infants: preliminary observations. *Pediatrics* 1985;75:217–25.
7. Jöbsis FF. Noninvasive, infrared monitoring of cerebral and myocardial oxygen sufficiency and circulatory parameters. *Science* 1977;198:1264.
8. Jöbsis FF, Keizer JH, LaManna JC, *et al*. Reflectance spectrophotometry of cytochrome aa₃ in vitro. *J Appl Physiol* 1977;43:858–72.
9. Rea PA, Crowe J, Wickramasinghe Y, Rolfe P. Noninvasive optical methods for the study of cerebral metabolism in the human newborn: a technique for the future? *J Med Eng Technol* 1985;9:160.
10. Schmidt S, Lenz A, Eilers H, Helledie N, Krebs D. Laserspectrophotometry in the fetus. *J Perinat Med* 1989;17:57.
11. Saling E. Die Untersuchungsmöglichkeiten des Kindes unter der Geburt (Einführung and Grundlagen). *Geburtshilfe Frauenheilkd* 1961;21:905.
12. Schmidt S, Langner K, Gesche J, Dudenhausen JW, Saling E. Der transkutan gemessene Kohlendioxydpartialdruck beim nicht hypoxischen Feten während der Geburt. *Geburtshilfe Frauenheilkd* 1983;43:538.
13. Weber T. Continuous fetal pH monitoring and neonatal Apgar score. *J Perinat Med* 1980;8:158.
14. Hochberg HM, Roby PV, Snell HM, Smith D, Chatterjee M. Continuous intrapartum fetal scalp tissue pH and ECG monitoring by a fiberoptic probe. *J Perinat Med* 1988;16(Suppl 1):71.
15. Huch A, Huch R. Fetal and maternal tcPO₂ monitoring. *Crit Care Med* 1981;9:694.
16. Severinghaus JW, Stafford M, Bradley AF. TcPCO₂ electrode design, calibration and temperature gradient problems. *Acta Anaesthesiol Scand* 1978;68:118.
17. Sturbois G, Uzan S, Rotten D, Breart G, Sureau C. Continuous subcutaneous pH measurement in human fetuses — correlation with scalp and umbilical blood pH. *Am J Obstet Gynecol* 1977;128:901.

DISCUSSION

Dr. Rosén: When evaluating a new variable such as cytochrome aa₃, there would be an advantage if you could compare it with another variable reflecting similar changes in intracellular energy status. My suggestion is that you carry on your experimental work but include hypoxanthine, which should reflect intracellular energy metabolism in the same way as cytochrome aa₃. Our own studies on the mature fetal lamb (1) have shown that measurable cerebral hypoxanthine production only occurs with a marked degree of asphyxia, since hypoxanthine is consumed by the brain during moderate asphyxia. I wonder therefore what degree of fetal asphyxia will be identified by the cytochrome aa₃ changes.

Dr. Schmidt: We do not really understand what is happening within the cell during asphyxia. My hope is that we can identify situations in the fetus in which changes in cytochrome would be more discriminating than those identifiable by other techniques such as cardiotocography.

Dr. Hope: I am concerned about the inaccuracy that may result because of the large fall in signal intensity with signal depth. By the time the signal has passed through 9 cm or so of maternal tissue very little of the reflected signal will represent anything to do with the fetal brain. I am also concerned by the lack of quantitation in your system. If you have a near-infrared source and the sensor is in a constant position, as when a cup is fitted onto the head, then you have an approximately constant path length and can get some comparability between readings from different fetuses. However, if the path length is completely unknown and variable, as it is with abdominal application, it produces major problems of quantitation.

Dr. Schmidt: Thank you. I did not mention this problem and I am glad it has been addressed. At present we cannot acquire absolute values, so we can only see relative changes. Clinicians must use the technique synchronously with the cardiotocograph, looking for relative changes.

Dr. Golbus: I agree that transcutaneous application is going to be necessary if this technique is to be widely used clinically. In answer to Dr. Hope's concern, I wonder why we could not have a second set of senders and receivers right next to the first set, but only measuring the thickness of the maternal tissues. The computer could then correct for the maternal tissue signal by simply subtracting it from the maternal plus fetal signal.

Dr. Schmidt: That is a very good point. This is something that Peter Rolf is examining and we know from ultrasound work that such techniques can be made to work.

Dr. Van Geijn: We all know that some particular areas of the brain are more susceptible to reduced flow or hypoxemia than others. How specific can this method be in this regard?

Dr. Schmidt: The scattering area is some 5 cm.

Dr. Dawes: The sampling time is 2 s. Why do you choose such a long time?

Dr. Schmidt: During the animal experiments we wanted an even longer sampling time of 10 s in order to correlate the different recorded variables.

Dr. Dawes: If you use a short laser pulse, could you get better discrimination?

Dr. Hope: No, as far as I know this is not possible. The speed of light is such that any gating is impracticle.

Dr. Dawes: In summary, you are sampling from a large block of tissue, larger than the fetal brain. We already know that there is a change in flow in different areas of the fetal brain depending on sleep states. So I don't think you can reliably tell what is going on until you can detect that change.

Dr. Schmidt: The aim must be to get smaller biological samples, but at present we are unable to focus the beam.

Dr. Dawes: Is there any problem with heat dissipation?

Dr. Schmidt: Not with this kind of energy. The mean energy is only 4 mW. I should mention that when pulse laser light is used the peaks of energy are much higher, but we still believe we are within the safety range because we work at wavelengths where the photon energy should be very low.

REFERENCE

1. Thiringer K, Blomstrand S, Hrbek A, Karlsson K, Kjellmer I. Cerebral arterio-venous difference for hypoxanthine and lactate during graded asphyxia in the fetal lamb. *Brain Res* 1982;239:107–17.

Perinatology, edited by Erich Saling,
Nestlé Nutrition Workshop Series, Vol. 26,
Nestec, Ltd., Vevey/Raven Press, Ltd.,
New York © 1992.

Clinical Validity of Fetal ECG Waveform Analysis

Karl G. Rosén, *S. Arulkumaran, †K. R. Greene, ‡H. Lilja,
§K. Lindecrantz, ¶H. Seneviratne, and C. Widmark

*Division of Perinatal Physiology, Department of Physiology and Paediatrics 1,
University of Göteborg, Sweden; *Department of Obstetrics and Gynecology, National
University of Singapore, Singapore; †Department of Obstetrics and Gynecology,
Freedomfield Hospital, Plymouth, United Kingdom; ‡Department of Obstetrics and
Gynecology, University of Göteborg, and §Department of Applied Electronics,
Chalmers University of Technology, Göteborg, Sweden; and ¶Department of
Obstetrics and Gynecology, University of Colombo, Sri Lanka*

Our ability to identify the fetuses at risk of intrapartum asphyxia depends on either monitoring the actual level of hypoxemia using biochemical means or, by different techniques, interpreting the reactions caused by hypoxemia. The fetal ability to adapt to hypoxemia involves multiple defense mechanisms. These consist primarily of cardiovascular compensation which increases blood flow to the most important organs—the brain, the heart, and the adrenals, as well as the placenta—and counteracts the decreasing oxygen content. A second line of defense is the metabolic compensatory mechanisms. This chapter presents data of the fetal reaction to hypoxemia as interpreted from ECG analysis.

During labor, the ECG signal is easily obtainable and additional information may be gathered without the need to change patient handling routines. Changes in the ECG waveform have been the subject of much clinical interest throughout the last 30 years (1,2). Throughout the past 10 years, this interest has been focused on detection of specific hypoxia-related phenomena (3).

BASIC RESEARCH—ST WAVEFORM

Since the initial experimental observations in 1972, there has been a continuous line of basic research to clarify some of the pathophysiological mechanisms involved in the elevation of the ST segment and T wave amplitude as a fetal response to hypoxia. In summary (Fig.1), the increase in T wave height, quantified by the ratio between T wave and QRS amplitudes (T/QRS ratio), occurs when the cardiovascular adaptation to hypoxia (increased coronary blood flow) is no longer sufficient. Myocardial metabolic adjustments are needed to cover for a negative energy balance.

Myocardial energy balance

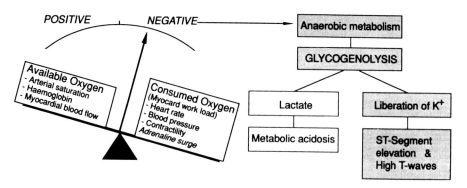

FIG. 1. A schematic presentation of the mechanisms involved in the appearance of ST segment elevation and high T waves. (Figure used with permission from Cinventa AB.)

Glycogenolysis, stimulated by adrenaline surge, becomes the most important source of energy and at the same time there is a change in membrane potential due to potassium release causing the ST elevation (4,5). Perhaps the best way of displaying these changes experimentally is during spontaneous labor in the chronically instrumented fetal sheep. Figure 2 gives an example of such a case where labor ended in fetal death at the time of delivery and a number of parameters were recorded in parallel with the ECG waveform. Eleven hours before fetal death the T/QRS ratio increased and during the last hour a further increase was noted with an increase in T/QRS ratio from 0.6 to 1.0. Figure 3 shows changes in cardiovascular parameters and somatosensory evoked EEG potentials during the last hours. Evoked potentials could serve as a measure of the ability of the fetal brain to operate during hypoxia (6) and it is obvious that from recordings like this, as well as from other data (7,8), ST waveform changes appear before loss of brain function. Figure 3 also indicates the capacity of the fetus to compensate for asphyxia with adequate brain signal processing in spite of marked acidosis. There are only a few minutes between the loss of cerebral activity and the last heart beat in this mature fetal lamb.

Further experimental work in the experimentally growth-retarded guinea pig fetus indicates the development of ST depression with a negative-positive T wave during hypoxemia. Thus, a "biphasic" ST waveform seems to be a most significant response.

ECG WAVEFORMS RECORDED FROM THE SCALP LEAD

All the animal experiments have used the precordial ECG lead which is optimal to identify all waveform components in the ECG. The QRS complex as well as the P wave are robust parameters, whereas the amplitude of the T wave is greatly influenced by the ECG vector. Lindecrantz *et al.* (9) have presented data to indicate

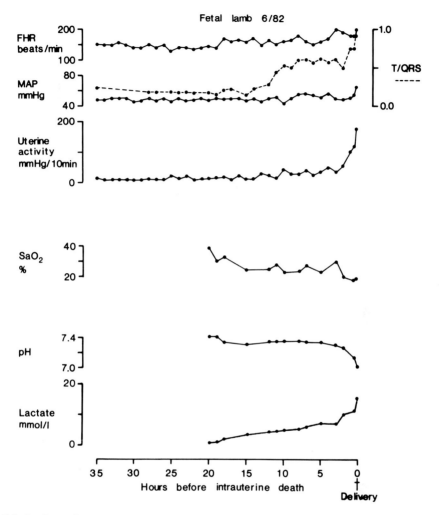

FIG. 2. Recordings from a chronically instrumented sheep fetus during spontaneous labor ending in fetal death at time of delivery. FHR, fetal heart rate; MAP, mean arterial pressure; SaO₂, oxygen saturation. Data modified from Rosén KG, *et al.* (7).

that the standard bipolar scalp lead (an exploring electrode inserted in the scalp with a reference electrode placed close by and in contact with the vaginal fluid) was only optimal in identifying T wave changes occurring in the horizontal $(x + z)$ plane of the fetal body. The x-axis has consistently been unable to detect changes in the T wave amplitude, which means that the standard scalp ECG used for cardiotocography (CTG) monitoring is not optimal for ST analysis. On the other hand, the y-axis, which identifies changes in the longitudinal plane of the fetal body, is optimal for detection of changes in T wave height. This y-lead is simply recorded by using

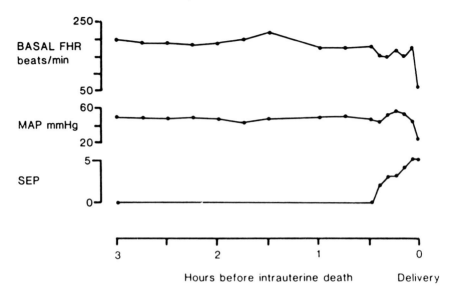

FIG. 3. Last 3 h of labor. Data from the same recording as in Fig. 2. Note the maintained somatosensory evoked response (SEP) until the last 20 min. SEP was quantified according to a scoring system where 0 = normal response, and 5 = no response at all. For further details see refs. 7 and 8.

a unipolar scalp lead. Our model for creating this unipolar scalp lead during labor is to place the reference electrode far away from the scalp, i.e., on the maternal thigh. Apart from increased sensitivity for changes in T wave configuration, there is also an increase in signal quality, due to less ECG baseline shift (10). This is not of minor importance as any further attempt to reduce this low frequency shift by signal filtering could seriously affect the low-frequency components of the ECG—the ST period (11,12). Furthermore, our experience with different scalp electrodes has consistently indicated that one helix scalp electrode gives the least baseline shift as well as the optimal signal amplitude.

APPROPRIATE TECHNOLOGY

There has been a continuous development in technology in the last 10 years with the aim of developing a robust, user-friendly monitor. Throughout this process, data have been collected using currently available technology. In our initial study (13), standard equipment was used (oscilloscope and Mingograph ECG-recorder) and with further development, a purpose-built microprocessor for ST-ANalysis (STAN) was constructed.

STAN—A CTG Monitor with ST Waveform Analysis

The ST analyzing system is displayed schematically in Fig. 4. The fetal ECG is picked up differentially between a one helix scalp electrode and a skin electrode

STAN

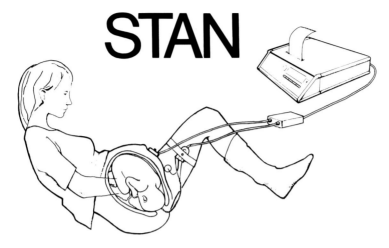

FIG. 4. A schematic presentation of the STAN system. Note that the only extra is a ordinary skin electrode placed on the maternal thigh. (Figure used with permission from Cinventa AB.)

placed on the maternal thigh. Both electrodes are connected to a patient isolating box (PIB), via an ECG clip connector. In the PIB the ECG signal is amplified and this unit also contains the necessary galvanic isolation between the patient and the rest of the system. The PIB also has an input connector for a uterine activity signal from an external toco transducer or an internal uterine pressure transducer. From the PIB, which is kept close to the patient, both toco and ECG signals are led to the main unit through a cable that can be of several meters' length.

The main unit, where most of the signal processing and the computations are performed, is furnished with a one-color printer plotter for data presentation, a graphic LC display and five push buttons for software control functions. Via a serial interface (RS 232) the signals can be presented to a personal computer for further processing and storage. The ECG signal from the PIB passes through an adaptive line frequency filter that eliminates 50 or 60 Hz interference in the signal. The bandwidth used for waveform analysis is 0.05–100 Hz and the signal is A to D converted at the rate of 500 Hz with a resolution corresponding to 8 bits. For further details of the system, see Rosén *et al.* (14).

Once the machine is connected to the patient and turned on, it automatically adjusts gain level and the processed data are presented on both the LC display and the printer/plotter. Fetal heart rate and toco activity are presented on the printer according to accepted standards for CTG monitors. The T/QRS ratios are also presented as a function of time, and every second minute an average fetal ECG complex is plotted (Fig. 5).

The Nottingham group, headed by M. Symonds, has developed a separate system of ECG time interval analysis (15). This system has been based on a minicomputer system with an ongoing effort to develop a microprocessor-based unit. The aim of the Nottingham system is to enable on-line assessment of a multitude of ECG parameters—time constants as well as alterations in waveforms. This approach has

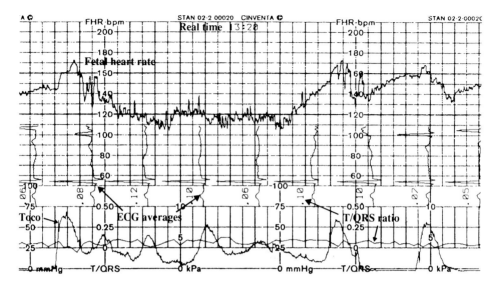

FIG. 5. An example of a STAN printout.

been fruitful as it has empirically, during labor, identified changes in the PR time constant which shortens during hypoxemia in spite of a lengthening of the RR (decreasing heart rate).

CLINICAL STUDIES—ST WAVEFORM

In the initial study (13) we were able to demonstrate, with simple technology, that it was possible to detect ST waveform changes during labor and these changes occurred independently of CTG changes. Furthermore, a linear relationship was found between T/QRS ratio and umbilical lactate levels. The number of patients in the study was small ($n = 46$) and no clinically asphyxiated babies were found. In a subsequent study (16) the first microprocessor version of STAN was tested with a continuous recording of T/QRS ratios using the group averaging technique. Only one fetus showed a T/QRS ratio >0.30 throughout the 2.5 h recording. Umbilical artery pH was 7.05 and lactate was 7.73 mmol/l with normal Apgar scores and neonatal outcome. There were two more fetuses with ST waveform changes lasting more than 30 min; both of these had CTG changes as well as high lactate and low pH values. There was one case with biphasic T waves showing a marked respiratory acidosis (pH 7.06). In eight cases blood was available for catecholamine analysis. A significant correlation, $r = 0.73$, $p < 0.05$, was found between adrenaline concentration and T/QRS ratio, but no correlation was found between noradrenaline and T/QRS. Both studies were small by their numbers and did not incorporate any child with clinical asphyxia, but they still provided information on the technology needed and some indications were found of a parameter, the T/QRS ratio, which might independently provide information of fetal response to hypoxia in labor.

With the need for a larger population of high-risk pregnancies, collaboration was started with the National University of Singapore and the University of Colombo, Sri Lanka. The first major data base on ST waveform analysis during labor using the STAN monitor has recently been collected (10,17), and the normal range of T/QRS ratios during labor in healthy fetuses was shown to be 0.15 ± 0.05 (mean ± 1 SD) (10). The ratio was found to be most stable during labor with an occasional increase during contraction, but this was not a regular finding as can be seen in Fig. 4.

The second study (17) is based on 201 deliveries, 25% at high risk. Cord artery pH and buffer balance together with Apgar scores were used as end points of perinatal asphyxia. During first stage of labor 45% had suspicious or abnormal heart rate traces, whereas only 27% had a baseline T/QRS ratio >0.25 (+2 SD). Twenty-seven operative deliveries were performed for fetal distress diagnosed on CTG findings, and in three of these the cord artery blood pH was <7.15. Among these 27 fetuses, 11 (41%) displayed elevated baseline T/QRS, which identified all fetuses with cord artery pH <7.15 and/or standard bicarbonate <15.0 mmol/l.

It was of special interest to correlate the reduction in buffering capacity of the fetal blood as identified by a standard bicarbonate <15.0 mmol/l with the increase in T wave amplitude. The normal ST waveform identified with a probability of 99.3% a fetus with normal buffering capacity. Five fetuses developed a metabolic acidosis (pH <7.15 and standard bicarbonate <15.0 mmol/l), all of whom showed high T/QRS ratios. Acute hypoxia emerging during second stage of labor was identified by rapid rise in T/QRS. There were three cases with a clinical diagnosis of asphyxia, all were identified by changes in T/QRS, and the lowest 5-min Apgar was 6. An evaluation test between T/QRS during first stage of labor and reduced buffer capacity in the cord artery blood showed a sensitivity of 94% and a specificity of 80%. Kappa index was 0.40.

CTG on its own did not reflect the acid-base status in cord artery. However, in the group of fetuses (five cases) with abnormal CTG and increased mean T/QRS, four had a low bicarbonate concentration and metabolic acidosis always occurred when there were changes in both ST waveform and CTG (Table 1). Thus, it seems possible to increase the specificity and positive predictive value by combining T/QRS with fetal heart rate.

The first independent trial on STAN has been performed by Murphy, Valente, and Johnson in Oxford (18). Their data are based on 86 recordings using a STAN prototype monitor which they found was robust and suitable for clinical application. Of the recordings, 97% were of a quality to allow ECG waveform analysis. Only one fetus developed clinical problems related to perinatal asphyxia, identified from metabolic acidosis in the cord artery and vein (cord artery pH 6.96, standard bicarbonate 13.6 mmol/l, standard base excess −16.0 mmol/l). Apgar scores were 2 and 7, with some respiratory distress during the neonatal period. This case revealed a high T/QRS ratio during first stage (mean T/QRS 0.31). During the end of the first

TABLE 1. *Relationship between fetal heart rate (FHR) and average T/QRS ratio during first stage of labor*

	T/QRS			
FHR	<0.25	0.26–0.49	>0.50	*n*
Normal	80 (*1:0*)[a]	21 (*5:0*)	0	101
Suspicious	43	23 (*7:3*)	0	66
Abnormal	10	5 (*4:2*)	0	15
n	133	49	0	182

[a] (*x:y*), *x* = number of cases with standard bicarbonate < 15.0 mmol/l; *y* = number of cases with pH < 7.15.

stage and in the second stage a "biphasic" ST waveform with a negative T wave component with ST segment depression occurred. The authors also analyzed the relationship between CTG, using Krebs intrapartum CTG score, and T/QRS ratio, and showed a significant relationship between high T/QRS values and low-scoring (abnormal) segments of the intrapartum CTG ($p<.01$).

Of the ongoing trials, the largest series of cases has been collected in Colombo. At the time of writing, 485 recordings have been analyzed, showing a success rate of 97% using the one helix scalp electrode. There has been one case of intrapartum death, which was monitored. Monitoring means heart rate from the STAN, but not ECG waveform for clinical management. This fetus was severely growth-retarded (birth weight 1.700 g at term) and displayed negative T waves. This pattern was already evident at the beginning of the 8-hour recording. Figure 6 shows the recording 1 h before fetal death demonstrating increasingly negative T waves. Figure 7 shows another recording lasting 20 min, in a full-term, appropriately grown fetus. The baseline bradycardia was noted in first stage and after a manual dilatation of the cervix a vacuum extractor was applied. The baby was delivered with Apgar scores of 2 and 5 and showed seizures at 24 hours after birth. The subsequent neonatal outcome was uneventful.

ONGOING TRIALS

Through the European Community concerted action project "New Methods for Perinatal Surveillance," a multicenter prospective study is now starting, involving 10 to 15 European perinatal centers. The ECG is collected "blind" and the purpose is to build a European ECG data base. STAN is used as an ordinary CTG monitor with a PC backup system for data handling and subsequent storing, which uses optical disks to handle the large amount of data generated. The plan is to collect the ECG in a format that will allow off-line analysis of all ECG-related parameters like power spectrum analysis of heart rate variability and time interval analysis. The latter is of special interest as the Nottingham group (15) has demonstrated the relevance of

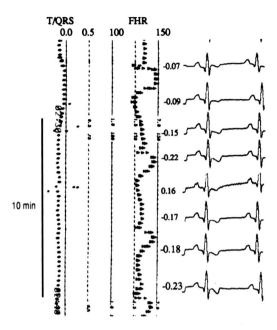

FIG. 6. Heart rates, T/QRS ratios, and fetal ECG averages recorded during labor in a severely growth-retarded fetus. The recording was obtained 1 hour before fetal death.

a change in correlation between PR and RR time constants with intrapartum hypoxia. Normally this correlation is positive, i.e., with increasing RR (lower heart rate) there is also an increase in PR but with hypoxia the PR shortens in spite of lengthening of RR and the correlation becomes negative. Sheep experimental data support this finding and there are now data (15,17) to indicate that by combining different aspects of the ECG one should be able to improve the diagnostic properties.

TENTATIVE MODEL FOR ST WAVEFORM ANALYSIS

On the basis of approximately 1,500 cases where ST waveform monitoring has been undertaken, together with our experience from the animal data base, there is a possibility of making a tentative model of the relationship between the ability of the fetus to react to hypoxia and the appearance of the ST waveform changes. Figure 8 summarizes this model, and the reaction of the fetus to hypoxia is separated into three groups:

1. Those with *intact* defense mechanisms
2. Those with *reduced* defense mechanisms
3. Those *lacking* defense mechanisms.

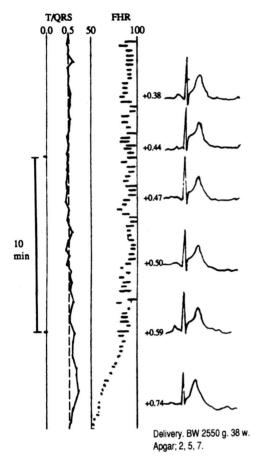

FIG. 7.   STAN recording in a case with neonatal seizures and perinatal asphyxia.

Intact Defense Mechanisms

These are the majority of fetuses, approaching 99%. Those fetuses have developed all the resources needed to handle asphyxia, including energy stores, optimal reactivity regarding the sympathetic system and catecholamine release, optimal receptor sensitivity, etc. This gives optimal hypoxia reactivity and full compensation over long periods of hypoxemia and also an ability to handle severe asphyxia. The occurrence of ST segment elevation and increase in T wave height signifies a situation in which glycogenolysis is occuring and an important defense mechanism is in operation. How could we then identify the point at which these mechanisms no longer fully support the fetus? At the moment the data indicate that such a situation can be identified by a combination of increasing and/or sustained high T/QRS ratio with signs of a reduced reactivity in the fetal heart rate pattern.

What is happening to the fetus when these patterns emerge? A case showing such marked changes is presented in Fig. 7. This baby responded to resuscitation and

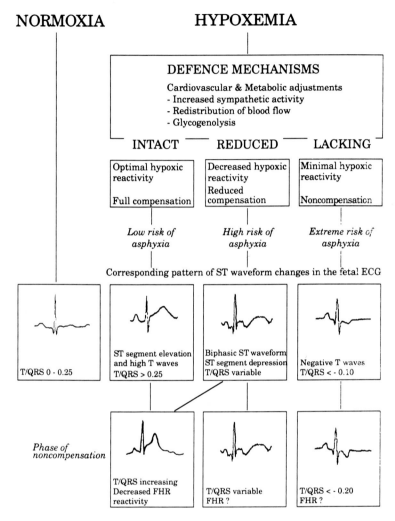

FIG. 8. A tentative model of interpretation of ST waveform and heart rate changes. (Figure used with permission from Cinventa AB.)

survived the neonatal period with only a short-lasting seizure 24 hours after birth. The Singapore data also tell us that the combination of elevated T waves and abnormal CTG will identify fetuses with a decreased buffer capacity but who are clinically normal at birth.

Reduced Defense Mechanisms

This is a situation that could be identified experimentally using the growth-retarded guinea pig model and subjecting these fetuses to hypoxemia. They are moderately growth-retarded which means that they survive labor but show a decrease in their hypoxic reactivity and ability to compensate. Their ability to maintain cellular integrity is curtailed and the risk for decompensation and asphyxia will increase. In his experimental work Carl Widmark has demonstrated "biphasic" ST waveform as a characteristic response to hypoxemia.

Biphasic T Wave

Clinically as well as experimentally the ST waveform shows "biphasic" T wave with a negative T wave component occurring together with a positive component. This pattern has only been recorded in a few cases but all of those have developed asphyxia, identified by metabolic acidosis base deficit >12 mmol/l), decrease in Apgar scores and neonatal problems (seizures or respiratory distress). It seems as though biphasic patterns may either be sustained throughout labor or develop into high T waves. The T/QRS ratio will vary but usually goes beyond 0.25 as the positive T wave will dominate.

CTG

The relationship with CTG has, so far, been one of parallel changes. It could be anticipated, however, that heart rate would not show distinct changes because there is still some reactivity and heart rate is poor when it comes to quantifying the reactive patterns. The incidence of these changes is probably on the order of 0.5–1%.

Lacking Defense Mechanisms

Here we have severely growth-retarded fetuses who may not be able to handle labor at all, probably due to the long-term stress. Reactivity to hypoxia is minimal and the risk of decompensation is imminent, leading to extreme risk of asphyxia. As there is no capacity to compensate by using metabolic mechanisms, the degree of metabolic acidosis might be less. It also seems likely that these fetuses could suffer permanent damage at a far lower degree of hypoxemia than would be the case with a fetus who was able to compensate. Due to the work in Colombo, we have been able to identify the pattern of negative T waves that seems to reflect this grossly adverse situation. This may be a unique piece of information obtainable only from ECG waveform analysis. It seems logical that an indicator of organ function should be able to signify a situation of extreme risk. Identifying such situations is of vital importance in the reduction of perinatal mortality and morbidity.

This model of ECG data interpretation during labor is presently tested in a randomized controlled trial that is taking place in Plymouth. The data obtained from the study of 600 cases show that ST and CTG monitoring in combination could reduce the rate of operative deliveries by more than 50% with no increased risk of perinatal asphyxia as compared with the use of CTG alone (K. R. Greene and J. Westgate, personal communication).

ACKNOWLEDGMENTS

This work was supported by the Swedish Medical Research Council (5654, 2591), the Swedish Board of Technical Development, Wilhelm & Martina Lundgrens Forskningsfond, the Expressen Perinatal Research Foundation, the Swedish Society of Medicine, and the First of Mayflower Annual Campaign for Children's Health.

REFERENCES

1. Larks SD. The abnormal fetal electrocardiogram: intrauterine fetal difficulty and fetal distress. *Obstet Gynecol* 1963;22:427–32.
2. Pardi G, Tucci E, Uderzo A, Zanini D. Fetal electrocardiogram changes in relation to fetal heart rate pattern during labor. *Am J Obstet Gynecol* 1974;118:243–6.
3. Greene KR. The ECG waveform. In: Whittle M, ed. *Baillier's clinical obstetrics and gynaecology*, vol 1. London: WB Saunders, 1987;131–55.
4. Rosén KG. Alterations in the fetal electrocardiogram as a sign of fetal asphyxia—experimental data with a clinical implementation. *J Perinat Med* 1986;14:355–63.
5. Rosén KG, Arulkumaran S, Thavarasah AS, et al. ST waveform analysis of the fetal ECG during labour—initial report of the STAN multicenter trial. In: Genser G, Marsál K, Svenningsen N, Lindström K, eds. *Fetal and neonatal physiological measurements* III. Malmö, Sweden: Flenhags Tryckeri, 1989;157–68.
6. Hrbek A, Karlsson K, Kjellmer I, Olsson T, Riha M. Cerebral reactions during intrauterine asphyxia in the sheep. II. Evoked electroencephalogram responses. *Pediatr Res* 1974;8:58–63.
7. Rosén KG, Lilja H, Hökegård KH, Kjellmer I. The relationship between cerebral cardiovascular and metabolic functions during labour in the lamb fetus. In: Jones CT, ed. *Symposium on the physiological development of the fetus and newborn.* London: Academic Press, 1985.
8. Rosén KG, Hrbek A, Karlsson K, Kjellmer I, Olsson T, Riha M. Changes in the ECG and somatosensory-evoked EEG responses during intrauterine asphyxia in the sheep. *Biol Neonate* 1976;30:95–101.
9. Lindecrantz K, Lilja H, Widmark C, Rosén KG. Fetal ECG during labour: a suggested standard. *J Biomed Eng* 1988;10:351–3.
10. Lilja H, Arulkumaran S, Ratnam SS, Rosén KG. Fetal ECG during labour: a presentation of a microprocessor system. *J Biomed Eng* 1988;10:348–50.
11. Greene KR. *Quantification of ST waveform changes of the fetal ECG and their relationship to asphyxia.* MD Thesis. Southampton: University of Southampton, 1983.
12. Lindecrantz K. *Processing of the fetal ECG: an implementation of a dedicated real time microprocessor system.* Technical report No 135. Gothenburg, Sweden: Chalmers University of Technology, 1983.
13. Lilja H, Greene KR, Karlsson K, Rosén KG. ST waveform changes of the fetal electrocardiogram during labour—a clinical study. *Br J Obstet Gynecol* 1985;92:611–7.
14. Rosén KG, Lindecrantz K. STAN — the Gothenburg model for fetal surveillance during labour by ST analysis of the fetal electrocardiogram. *Clin Phys Physiol Meas* 1989;10(Suppl 10):51–6.
15. Murray HG. The fetal electrocardiogram: current clinical developments in Nottingham. *J Perinat Med* 1986;14:399.
16. Lilja H. Microprocessor based waveform analysis of the fetal electrocardiogram during labor. *Int J Gynecol Obstet* 1989;30:109–16.
17. Arulkumaran S, Lilja H, Lindecrantz K, Ratnam SS, Thavarasah AS, Rosén KG. Fetal ECG waveform analysis should improve fetal surveillance in labour. *J Perinat Med* 1990;18:13–22.
18. Murphy KW, Valente J, Johnson P. Clinical evaluation of fetal ECG monitoring in labour. *Br J Obstet Gynaecol* (in press).

DISCUSSION

Dr. Dawes: In your presentation you mentioned a randomized controlled trial. What is the basis for clinical management in the group of fetuses where the STAN monitor is used?

Dr. Rosén: In this study we are comparing standard management, including CTG and fetal blood sampling in one leg of the study with CTG, and fetal blood sampling and ST waveform analysis in the other. Using the ST waveform we have one variable that is independent of heart rate. The aim of the trial is to test whether ST waveform could add to clinical management, reducing the number of operative interventions without increasing the risk of intrapartum asphyxia. In the protocol it is stated that with a normal ST waveform, blood sampling should be postponed until the trace becomes persistently abnormal. If there is a preterminal fetal heart rate pattern, operative delivery is performed. A normal ST waveform means that interference can be delayed. When there is a normal fetal heart rate with a T/QRS ratio between 0.25 and 0.5 we just observe closely. When both variables identify changes, further information is needed from fetal blood sampling. If there are marked changes, immediate delivery is indicated.

Normally the T/QRS ratio is stable during labor, which means that a long-term trend with a persistent increase in the ratio signifies that the fetus needs additional energy from stored myocardial glycogen.

On the extremely rare occasions when there are biphasic T waves, fetal blood sampling is performed even if there is a normal fetal heart rate pattern. I believe that this situation signifies a fetus lacking the ability to compensate for asphyxia and rapidly approaching the stage of decompensation.

Dr. Saling: When do you think this method of monitoring should be considered? After all, it is a traumatic procedure requiring the introduction of the electrode and sometimes the rupture of the membranes.

Dr. Rosén: The advantage of the ECG waveform analysis is that we do not need to change our patient-handling procedures, since a scalp electrode is already required for cardiotocographic analysis during labor. Naturally it would be a great advantage if we could do waveform analysis before labor, using the transabdominally recorded ECG. Unfortunately I do not think this is possible because of the vectorcardiographic aspects. It is possible to obtain the ECG waveform analysis antenatally via a needle used for transfusing the fetus, though unfortunately the cord does not seem to give an ECG signal.

Dr. Marini: Changes in the T wave indicate that the metabolism of the heart is impaired; this can be either because of hypoxia or because of impairment of the coronary circulation. Do you know which heart chamber you are actually reading?

Dr. Rosén: The unipolar system provides a stable signal that is independent of the position of the head. It should identify the Y vector which reflects events in both ventricles.

Dr. Marini: When you did your study in animals, you probably followed the animals until death. Did you find any case of ventricular fibrillation before death or did the animals all die with cardiac arrest? I ask this because it is very uncommon for neonates to die with ventricular fibrillation, but in our work with the isolated neonatal heart (1) it was very common to induce ventricular fibrillation. It sounds as though the innervation of the heart will protect the neonatal heart from VF.

Dr. Rosén: We have not found ventricular fibrillation in our experiments, though sometimes there has been atrioventricular block.

Dr. Dawes: In the trial you are contemplating in primates, I think you said that you were going to combine ST segment analysis with a visual analysis of fetal heart rate. However, the visual analysis of fetal heart rate patterns is suspect and the Krebs score worse than suspect — it is positively misleading. This score requires selection of an identifiable piece of the trace in which 50% is "characteristic." This is not a logical prescription. The Krebs score has five variables, each scored from 0 to 2, so the maximum is 10. One of the variables concerns fetal heart rate, the second concerns the presence or absence of decelerations. The three other variables relate to fetal heart rate variability, including decelerations, zero crossing frequency, and amplitude. This score therefore gives an excessive weighting to heart rate variability, without justification. In the present state of knowledge such scores are best avoided. My advice in planning this proposed study in primates is to avoid scoring the cardiotocogram by visual analysis.

Dr. Rosén: We are not going to use the Krebs score. At the same time we must accept that visual analysis of the CTG is the present standard and we want to take the development step by step toward more objective analysis.

Dr. Dawes: Would Professor Saling agree with the statement that CTG visual analysis is the present standard?

Dr. Saling: When evaluating the CTG we use the Hammacher score, but this is also a complicated procedure. Up to now nothing better has been possible. But perhaps now with computer evaluation we shall be more objective.

Dr. Dawes: May I ask about the PR:RR ratio you mentioned? This was from a study by Henry Murray in Nottingham. I wonder whether you have any explanation of the curious relationship he described.

Dr. Rosén: The alteration in the relationship between the PR and RR time intervals was first observed by Henry Murray in his evaluation of approximately 300 labor recordings. The Nottingham group has used the correlation between the two time intervals as a way to identify the abnormal response of a shortening in the PR with a lengthening in the RR. A normal PR:RR correlation seemed to indicate that the fetus was healthy and had a normal acid-base status. By combining ST segment analysis with PR analysis they were able to identify fetuses with cord acidemia.

We have started experimental work to try to identify the pathophysiological mechanisms for the changes in the PR:RR correlation. A change in the relationship can be induced experimentally by a period of hypoxia lasting between one and 20 min. Under these circumstances, ST waveform and PR:RR changes occur in parallel. However, β-adrenoceptor stimulation, which causes increased T wave height, does not alter the PR-RR correlation. We are currently using the STAN monitor linked to a common PC for data collection in a multicenter study; it is hoped this will create a data base of ECG complexes that will allow us to investigate different ECG-related variables during labor, such as ST waveform, time constants, and power spectrum analysis of fetal heart rate variability.

Dr. Marini: Pardi and Brambati have analyzed the lengths of the various segments of the fetal ECG. They found in a severely damaged fetus with erythroblastosis that duration was much more indicative of lesions than the height of the waves. I believe that if you do not know precisely where the signal is coming from it is more reliable to work on duration.

In one of your cases you showed a long wave in the QT segment, like an afterpotential. This could be important in discriminating between altered repolarization because of electrolyte imbalance and altered perfusion under the papillary muscle, which is one of the major causes of neonatal cardiac problems.

Have you found any cases of wandering pacemaker? This is very common in the neonatal age group and could explain the varying PR length.

Dr. Rosén: The change in the PR interval that occurs with acute asphyxia and bradycardia is a shortening without a marked change in P wave configuration. In the preterminal trace you may see an independent lengthening of the PR interval without change in P wave configuration, in which case a wandering pacemaker could explain the finding, as you suggest. The possibility of discriminating between electrolyte imbalance and ischemia from changes in QT sounds interesting. However, the QT interval is hard to define as the end of the T wave may not be distinct. Intracellular electrolyte disturbance is the most likely explanation of the ST changes, since fetal myocardial performance and coronary blood flow are well maintained during hypoxemia in a term fetus.

REFERENCE

1. Marini A, *et al.* Studies of myocardial metabolism in isolated newborn lamb heart. *Am It Ost Med Perin* 1979;100:16–26.

Perinatology, edited by Erich Saling,
Nestlé Nutrition Workshop Series, Vol. 26,
Nestec, Ltd., Vevey/Raven Press, Ltd.,
New York © 1992.

Clinical Aspects of Infections as a Cause of Prematurity: "A Continuum of Risk"

Calvin J. Hobel

Division of Maternal-Fetal Medicine, Cedars-Sinai Medical Center, 8700 Beverly Boulevard, Los Angeles, California 90048–0750, USA

One of several high priorities in clinical obstetrical research is the determination of the proportion of preterm deliveries caused by infection. If infection can be shown with a high degree of certainty to be a significant cause, and if the mechanisms are understood, a safe therapeutic scheme can be proposed to reduce the incidence of preterm birth.

Most infections have a prodromal phase: this premonitory phase is now referred to as a preclinical or "silent" infection. In order to understand more clearly the role of infection in clinical obstetrics, we must begin at an early stage. This chapter will focus on the continuum of risk from the silent stage of infection to the symptomatic phases, from the point of view of a clinical disease and from a mechanistic point of view.

SUBCLINICAL INFECTIONS

The major debate today is about whether infection precedes and initiates preterm labor and/or premature rupture of the membranes, or whether it is an associated event. Several years ago our group considered clinical infections as a significant contributor only at later stages in the pathophysiology of preterm labor (1). Figure 1 indicates that clinical infections occur during the symptomatic stages (Stage III A and B) of preterm labor. What is the current evidence for the role of subclinical infections (Stage II) in increasing the likelihood of preterm delivery or premature rupture of the membranes? We shall explore the risk factors associated with infection which are present before and during pregnancy.

Role of Infection Prior to Pregnancy

Only recently has prepregnant genital tract infection been considered an early cause of asymptomatic bacterial colonization of the uterine cavity. Toth *et al.* (2)

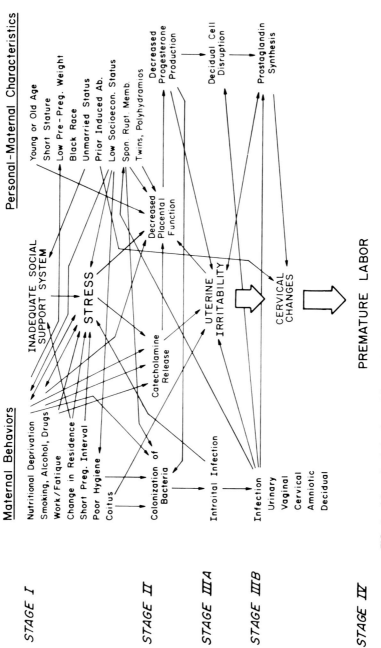

FIG. 1. A hypothesis for the multifactorial etiology of preterm labor. Stages I and II are considered silent or asymptomatic, whereas Stages III A and B are associated with clinical symptoms (1).

TABLE 1. *Risk factors for infection*

Prepregnancy
  History of septic abortion (2)
  History of pelvic inflammatory disease (3)
  History of intrauterine contraceptive device (3)
  Multiple sex partners (3)
  Presence of antisperm antibodies (3)
  History of pregnancy loss (3)
Pregnancy
  Maternal age (3,4)
  Number of pathogenic bacterial species at first visit (3)
  History of pregnancy loss (3)
  Asymptomatic bacteriuria (5–7)
  Sickle cell trait (8)
  Low social class (4,9)
  High parity (4)

Reference numbers in parentheses.

in 1986, reported a significant association between antibiotic therapy for septic abortions and subsequent pregnancy outcomes. They proposed that a subclinical infection persists in the endometrium and during a subsequent pregnancy, with its concomitant immune suppression, there is a persistence of the infection with a high probability of its evolution into a clinically important condition.

Risk Factors

If prepregnancy events are important, then what information is available on the role of risk factors in identifying patients at risk? More recently, Toth *et al.* (3) identified four significant risk factors associated with preterm birth and premature rupture of the membranes (Table 1). When these risk factors were entered into a logistic regression analysis, maternal age, numbers of pathogenic bacterial species, and history of pregnancy loss were still found to be significant. Their conclusion was that preexisting infection of the uterine cavity is a predisposing factor in preterm delivery.

Asymptomatic Bacteriuria During Pregnancy

The average incidence of asymptomatic bacteriuria in pregnancy is 5.1%, with a range of 3.8–9.7% (10). The incidence is similar in the pregnant and nonpregnant population; however, in pregnancy the incidence of symptomatic urinary tract infection is approximately three times that of the nonpregnant population (11,12). The increased risk of developing symptomatic infection in pregnancy is probably secondary to the urinary tract changes that occur, leading to stasis. It is also possible that some bacteria, such as the coliform bacilli, grow more rapidly in the urine of pregnant women than in that of nonpregnant controls (13).

Risk of Pyelonephritis

The risk of asymptomatic bacteriuria is considerable. Untreated women have on the average a 30% (range is 23–42%) risk of developing acute pyelonephritis, whereas the general incidence is <2% (10). Women who are treated have a risk of developing acute pyelonephritis of less than 5% (5).

Risk of Preterm Labor and Low Birth Weight

Kass (5) in 1962 was the first to note a very high prevalence of prematurity and perinatal mortality in infants of bacteriuric women (5). This was quickly reconfirmed by Kincaid-Smith and Bullen (6) in Australia in 1965. Kass also showed that both of these risks were significantly diminished when the bacteriuria was treated, although this was not confirmed by Kincaid-Smith and Bullen. These studies resulted in a considerable interest in the early diagnosis of asymptomatic bacteriuria. Between 1960 and 1971 there were 19 studies on the subject, of which only six showed a significant relationship between asymptomatic bacteriuria and the incidence of preterm delivery and low birth weight (7). Recently, Romero *et al.* (7) applied meta-analysis to examine the relationships between asymptomatic bacteriuria and preterm delivery and low birth weight. They classified reports according to study design into cohort studies and randomized treatment trials. Meta-analysis of cohort studies showed that untreated asymptomatic bacteriuria significantly increases the rates of both preterm delivery and low birth weight. The analysis of clinical trials showed that antibiotic treatment significantly reduced the risk of low birth weight. This careful analysis of the available clinical trials clearly indicates that antibiotic treatment of asymptomatic bacteriuria is effective in reducing the occurrence of low birth weight. The pathogens most frequently isolated from bacteriuric women are listed in Table 2. The species in this list are different from those identified by Toth *et al.* (3) in the cervix in first trimester pregnancies.

Risk Factors

Factors associated with a high incidence of asymptomatic bacteriuria are shown in Table 1 (8,9,14,15).

CLINICAL INFECTIONS

Vaginal-Cervical Colonization During Pregnancy

Very little is known about the time course between colonization of pathogens and the appearance of clinical symptoms meeting criteria for the diagnosis of vaginitis and the occurrence of preterm labor or premature rupture of the membranes (3,16).

TABLE 2. *Most frequently isolated pathogens in clinical infections*

Bacteriuric women (11)	Cervical-vaginal flora (asymptomatic) (3,16,17)	Vaginitis-cervicitis (16–18,22,25)	Preterm labor/delivery (28–31)
Escherichia coli · · · · · · · · · ·	·*E. coli*		
Klebsiella pneumoniae · · · · · ·	·*Kl. pneumoniae*		
Proteus mirabilis	Staph. aureus		
Pseudomonas aeruginosa	Stap. epidermidis		
Enterobacter cloacae	Strep. faecalis		
Enterobacter aerogenes	Strep. viridans		
Staphylococcus saprophyticus			
Enterococcus			
Group B β-hemolytic streptococcus · · · · · · · · · ·	·Group B streptococci · · · ·	·Group B streptococci	Group B streptococci
	Peptococcus spp.		
	Peptostreptococcus spp.		
	Clostridium		
	Bacteroides spp. · · · · · · ·	·Bacteroides spp. · · · · ·	·Bacteroides spp.
	Gardnerella · · · · · · · · ·	·Gardnerella · · · · · · ·	·Gardnerella
	Gonococcus · · · · · · · · ·	·Gonococcus · · · · · · ·	·Gonococcus
	Chlamydia · · · · · · · · · ·	·Chlamydia · · · · · · · ·	·Chlamydia(?)
	Trichomonas · · · · · · · ·	·Trichomonas · · · · · ·	·Trichomonas
		Candida albicans	
	Mycoplasma ·		·Mycoplasmas(?)
	Ureaplasma ·		·Ureaplasma(?)

· · · · · · · · · · · · · · ·, Pathogens shared by clinical infections.

Minkoff *et al.* (16) carried out a prospective study of vaginal flora by culturing 250 apparently asymptomatic patients early in pregnancy and relating their outcome to the presence or absence of various organisms. They found that patients who had *Trichomonas vaginalis* or *Bacteroides sp.* were more likely subsequently to experience premature rupture of the membranes, and those with *Ureaplasma urealyticum* more frequently began preterm labor. These authors cautiously interpreted their results by stating that a positive culture early in pregnancy may be noncausal or indirectly causal. Subsequent follow-up screening of these patients would be necessary to find a true correlation between the presence of these organisms and preterm birth or premature rupture of the membranes. As can be determined from Table 2, the pathogens found in the cervix and vagina of asymptomatic women are different from those of bacteriuric women but similar to those implicated in vaginitis, cervicitis, and preterm labor.

Vaginitis-Cervicitis

Vaginal discharge is the most frequent gynecologic complaint and it accounts for 7% of all patient visits to the obstetrician gynecologist (17). The diagnostic categories of vaginitis are: nonspecific, 40–50%; candidiasis, 20–30%; and trichomoniasis, 20–30%. In the normal nonsymptomatic patient there is a large number of microorganisms, many of which have pathogenic potential. However, the presence of lactobacilli is vital for restructuring the growth of other bacteria, primarily by maintaining a low vaginal pH. The mechanisms causing a change in the complex interrelationship between microorganisms is not well understood. Symptomatic vaginitis is most often secondary to an overgrowth of *Candida albicans* and *Gardnerella vaginalis* and also of sexually transmitted organisms such as *Trichomonas* or *Neisseria gonorrhoeae*. Cervicitis is considered to be an entity distinct from vaginitis (17). Approximately 25% of patients with vaginal discharge have cervicitis. The only known specific causes of cervicitis are *Neisseria gonorrhoeae, Chlamydia trachomatis*, and *Mycoplasma hominis*. There is increasing evidence that cervical and vaginal infection may cause a significant proportion of preterm deliveries.

Bacterial Vaginosis (Nonspecific Vaginitis)

As noted above, this diagnosis is made in about 50% of patients who complain of vaginal discharge, the associated organisms being *Gardnerella vaginalis* and *Bacteroides sp*. A prospective study by Gravett *et al.* (18) showed a significant association between premature rupture of the membranes, preterm labor, and amniotic infection in women who met criteria for the diagnosis of bacterial vaginitis. Nineteen percent of 534 pregnant women were found to have bacterial vaginosis. These same investigators, in a matched case-control study of patients with subclinical amniotic fluid infections, found a fourfold increase in the risk of premature labor in patients with this diagnosis (19). Even though Minkoff *et al.* (16) found that 31.8% of 233 prenatal patients had clinical criteria for nonspecific vaginitis they did not find an association with preterm labor. However, they did find a significantly increased incidence of *Bacteroides* isolation in those who delivered preterm, which is correlated with bacterial vaginosis.

Trichomonas Vaginalis

Early studies did not associate trichomoniasis with the risk of low birth weight (20). It is known that the organism may cause inflammation. Recently Minkoff found trichomonads in approximately 15% of prenatal patients, and these women were significantly more likely to have premature rupture of the membranes (16).

Vaginal Candidiasis

Candidiasis is the third most common vaginal infection during pregnancy and there is no apparent association with preterm birth or premature rupture of the membranes. The mechanisms by which the vagina is colonized with candida is not well understood. It appears that candida species are opportunistic pathogens that flourish only when the normal flora is altered. Progesterone receptors have been identified in the cytosol of *Candida albicans* which may explain the increased incidence of symptomatic disease observed in pregnancy (21). It is not known whether the recovery of this organism in up to approximately one-third of patients has any clinical significance with reference to preterm birth.

Chlamydia Trachomatis

Cervical infection with *Chlamydia trachomatis* has been associated with preterm labor, premature rupture of the membranes, and low birth weight (18,22). However, some studies have not supported this association (23,24). The reasons for these different findings are not clear. From my review of these papers, the selection of patients by risk factors, the timing of the first culture, and the reassessment as to recurrence are all issues that determine the final associations between positive results and poor perinatal outcome.

Neisseria Gonorrhoeae

The incidence of gonococcal infection in pregnant women ranges from 2.5% to 7.3% (25,26). Handsfield *et al.* (25) were the first to direct our attention toward gonococcal infection as a cause of preterm delivery and premature rupture of the membranes. These investigators observed a significantly greater incidence of *Neisseria gonorrhoeae* isolated from orogastric aspirates in women with preterm labor and premature rupture of the membranes than in a group without these complications. Their findings were consistent with the concept of "amniotic infection syndrome" proposed by Blanc 14 years earlier (27). These studies formed the basis for initiating the study of infection as a cause of these two major complications in obstetrics.

Mycoplasma Species

The role of *Mycoplasma species* in poor pregnancy outcome has been reviewed by Romero and Mazor (28). The rate of isolation of *Mycoplasma hominis* from cervicovaginal fluid was found to vary between 5% and 49% whereas that of *M. urealyticum* was higher, at 44% to 81%. After a careful review of over 17 publications these investigations came to the conclusion that only one randomized clinical trial (29), in which colonized women were treated with erythromycin, was associated with a lower prevalence of low birth weight infants. A second study, by Kundsin *et al.* (30), suggested a positive association between histologic chorioamnionitis and the isolation of *Ureaplasma urealyticum* (30). Thus at best there is little to suggest that cervical-vaginal colonization with mycoplasmas is a significant cause of either low birth weight or prematurity (31).

Cystitis/Pyelonephritis

This is one area of the spectrum of clinical infections in pregnant women that has received little recent attention. The linkage between asymptomatic bacteriuria and pyelonephritis is quite clear; little has been mentioned, however, about the likelihood of the occurrence of cystitis in patients who have asymptomatic bacteriuria (32).

Cystitis occurs in approximately 1.3–3.4% of pregnant patients (4,33). It is characterized by lower urinary tract symptoms (urinary urgency, frequency, dysuria, and suprapubic discomfort), the absence of systemic symptoms, and a positive urine culture. According to Harris and Gilstrap (33) cystitis in pregnancy is a distinct clinical syndrome different from both asymptomatic bacteriuria and pyelonephritis. Patients who develop cystitis have a 26% incidence of positive asymptomatic urine screens as compared to 80% of those who develop pyelonephritis. Likewise, the incidence of recurrence is only 17% compared to 33% for asymptomatic bacteriuria and 75% for pyelonephritis. It is very clear that cystitis may occur as a newly acquired complication of pregnancy, not highly associated with prior positive screening, and it has a low recurrence rate. The only reports associating cystitis with preterm labor or premature rupture of the membranes are by Mimouni *et al.* (34) in a group of insulin-dependent diabetic women. However, this study combined cystitis and vaginitis to form "urogenital infection" as the diagnostic category.

Acute pyelonephritis occurs in 1–2% of pregnant patients (32). Approximately 70–80% of patients who develop acute pyelonephritis during pregnancy have a prior history of asymptomatic bacteriuria. As noted earlier, the treatment of asymptomatic bacteriuria significantly reduces the risk of pyelonephritis. In the early 1960s Kass (5) showed that untreated women with asymptomatic bacteriuria had a high risk of developing pyelonephritis and when the condition was treated, not only was pyelonephritis prevented but the incidence of prematurity and low birth weight was also reduced. The association between preterm delivery and pyelonephritis is complex. It is most likely that the onset of preterm labor associated with pyelonephritis comes about by two different mechanisms, though these may be related. One mechanism is via the release of an endotoxin from bacteria in the bladder and kidney causing increased myometrial contractility (35). A second mechanism is via an associated ascending vaginal infection with necrosis of the decidua, release of lipases and prostaglandin production, also affecting uterine contractility (28). Thus in some cases preterm labor may not be caused directly by pyelonephritis. Gilstrap *et al.* (36) noted that delivery of low birth weight infants occurred exclusively in patients who had premature labor in association with acute pyelonephritis.

Amnionitis, Clinical and Subclinical

Maternal pyrexia has been the hallmark for the diagnosis of clinical chorioamnionitis; however, pyrexia is a late sign since infection within the amniotic cavity can be present with normal body temperature. The standard criteria used for the diagnosis of *clinical amnionitis* are maternal fever $\geq 37.8°C$ (100°F) plus two or more of the following: leukocytosis ($\geq 15,000$ per mm^3 with a shift to the left in the differential), maternal pulse >100 beats per min, fetal tachycardia ≥ 160 beats per min, and/or uterine tenderness (37). At the present time *subclinical amnionitis* is defined as the presence of a positive culture in the absence of the signs of clinical amnionitis (38). The combined incidence of these two clinical entities is between 0% and 25.8% (39). In 1977 Bobitt and Ledger were the first to provide evidence that amniotic fluid analysis in patients in preterm labor was positive for bacteria prior to the development of signs of maternal infection. This ushered in the concept of "subclinical" amnionitis (40,41). A subsequent study by Bobitt *et al.* (42) confirmed this finding and reported a 25% incidence of amniotic fluid infection in patients in preterm labor, and of these 75% were subclinical. These early reports led to several studies to determine the incidence of positive cultures (41–43). Wahbeh *et al.* (43) identified a subgroup of patients with extreme prematurity at highest risk of being colonized. This finding was consistent with the report from Naeye and Peters (44) whose analysis of the collaborative perinatal project data identified a peak incidence of amniotic fluid infections in the early pregnancy as a cause of perinatal deaths.

As more investigators begin to focus on subclinical intraamniotic infections, several important observations have been made. Hameed *et al.* (45) recognized that markers of infection (maternal C-reactive protein and amniotic fluid white cell count, gram stain, and culture) were significantly more common in cases that were refractory to tocolysis. These data indicated that the more difficult preterm labors may be due to infections that had reached the amniotic cavity. These data could support the concept that preterm labor due to milder infections in the decidual space or membranes, without invasion into the amniotic cavity, might be easier to inhibit with tocolytic therapy. Other studies have not been able to identify a high incidence of asymptomatic infections in women in preterm labor (46,47). The differences observed in these studies may be related to the differences used to define preterm labor, or to different population demographics, microbiologic techniques, and thresholds required for performing amniocentesis. This disparity between investigations makes it difficult to justify amniocentesis for microbiological evaluation of asymptomatic women with intact membranes and preterm labor.

There has been an ongoing controversy as to whether subclinical intra-amniotic infection or ascending type infection cause premature rupture of the membranes. There are some data to suggest that subclinical intra-amniotic infection can lead to premature rupture of the membranes. Leigh and Garite (48), who studied the value of amniocentesis in the management of premature labor with intact membranes, found that in all those who subsequently had premature rupture of the membranes positive cultures were present. In a study on the relationship between premature rupture of the membranes and fetal immunoglobulin production, Cederquist *et al.* (49) showed that fetuses from mothers with premature rupture of the membranes had significantly higher immunoglobulin levels than those of a control group. They found two patterns of infection. In a first group the peak immunoglobulin level occurred between 1 and 12 h after rupture of the membranes, while a second group peaked after 72 h. They hypothesized that in the first group the peak suggested that the infection was present before the membranes ruptured. There is thus considerable evidence to support the role of asymptomatic infection as a cause of preterm labor with and without premature rupture of the membranes. The pathogens identified in these patients are similar to those cultured from the vagina and cervix of asymptomatic and symptomatic women (vaginitis-cervicitis) (Table 2).

THE PATHOPHYSIOLOGY OF INTRAUTERINE INFECTION

Currently little attention is being directed toward understanding the mechanisms by which infection reaches the amniotic cavity. Romero and Mazor (28) carefully described the pathways for intrauterine infection. They concluded that indirect evidence indicates that the most common pathway is the ascending route, as opposed to the hematogenous route, or retrograde seeding via the fallopian tubes, or accidental introduction during intrauterine procedures. However, the investigations cited did not attempt to pursue the mechanisms by which organisms ascend through the cervix. If progress is to be made in the prevention of preterm birth, then investigations into these mechanisms must be pursued, since specific interventions to reduce or prevent bacteria from entering the uterus would be more efficacious than treating asymptomatic or symptomatic infections with antimicrobial agents.

Ascending Route of Infection

The mechanism by which bacteria pass the cervical barrier from the vagina into the uterus is of primary importance. The factors involved have not been clearly described. After an extensive review of the literature, I can propose a possible mechanism. For pelvic inflammatory disease the mechanisms by which infectious agents may spread from the lower to the upper genital tract have been described by Keith *et al.* (50). Three potential mechanisms have been described: trichomonads as vectors, sperm as vectors, and passive transport.

Trichomonads and Sperm as Vectors

There are data to suggest that both trichomonads and sperm act as vectors in pelvic inflammatory disease (50). Whether they play an important role in ascending infection in pregnancy remains to be studied; however, there is indirect evidence to support the fact that sperm may act as a vector. Bacteria are known to attach to sperm at both high and low bacterial concentrations (51). Bacteria have also been shown to attach to and invade the chorioamniotic membranes (52). Naeye and Ross (53) studied a clinic population in South Africa and found that premature delivery was four times more frequent in patients who had coitus. They observed a peak frequency of chorioamnionitis limited to the extraplacental membranes when labor and delivery took place within 2 days of the last coitus. This was only true when coitus occurred without a condom. Orgasm may also play a role: spontaneous rupture of the membranes occurred twice as frequently when there was recent coitus with orgasm than in patients with coitus without orgasm.

Passive Transport of Pathogens

Interest in the role of this mechanism stems from the early observations of Beck (54) in 1874, who showed that the rapid transport of sperm into the cervix and uterus cannot be accounted for entirely by sperm motility. The concept of active suction by the uterus during coitus was proposed by Heape (55) in 1898. During the 1930s, numerous studies using various techniques were performed in animal models to study sperm transport. This subject was reviewed by Noyes *et al.* in (56) 1958, but a sucking action of the uterus could not be confirmed. In the same year, Hartman (57) reviewed the subject and proposed that sperm migration must be dependent upon the muscular action of the female genital tract.

A breakthrough in this area of investigation occurred in 1960 when Bickers (58) demonstrated in human subjects that, in the absence of uterine contractions, the ascent of sperm in the human uterus was impossible. After placing carbon particles in the vagina prior to abdominal hysterectomy, Egli and Newton (59) observed carbon particles in the tubes within 30 min when oxytocin was administered. They concluded that contractions of the uterus were important for transporting the carbon particles into the uterus. The precise mechanical relationships that allow the passage of substances into the uterus was not established until Fox *et al.* (60) using a radiotelemetry device, studied the interrelationship between vaginal and uterine pressures during and after coitus. They identified a final negative pressure following female orgasm that could effect a sucking action of cervical mucus and entrapped sperm into the uterus.

The common denominator from studies on sperm migration in the nonpregnant women appears to be uterine contractility. Could uterine activity, as an active transport mechanism in pregnant women, cause the aspiration of cervical mucus and potential pathogens into the lower uterine segment and set the stage for a subclinical infection and possibly for clinical infection? We are currently studying this active transport mechanism, which is most plausible since excessive uterine activity is thought to precede preterm labor and premature rupture of the membranes (61). It is well recognized that important physiologic and anatomic changes occur in the uterus with the onset of labor. Reynolds (62) has described an increase in uterine myometrial tension in the fundus that exceeds the tension in the lower uterine segment. The result is a thinning of the lower segment and a gathering in of the myometrium. Thus there may be a passive mechanical aspiration of tissue components into the uterus together with contaminated material, setting the stage for subclinical infection between the uterine wall and the chorioamniotic membranes. I have referred to this as a squeeze (contraction), pull (suction) action that occurs because the cervix is anchored to the pelvis by the various ligaments, producing a zone of adhesion to allow this anatomical change to take place (Fig. 2). In support of both active and passive changes in the uterus it has been recently shown by de Vries *et al.* (63), using endovaginal real-time ultrasound, that rhythmic myometrial contractions of the inner myometrial third in pregnant and nonpregnant women are the rule rather than the exception. The majority of the uterine activity was retrograde, with

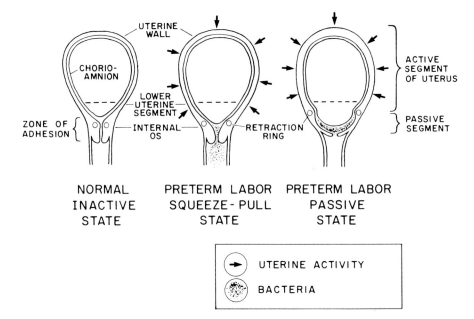

NORMAL
INACTIVE
STATE

PRETERM LABOR
SQUEEZE-PULL
STATE

PRETERM LABOR
PASSIVE
STATE

UTERINE ACTIVITY

BACTERIA

FIG. 2. Mechanism for ascending route of intrauterine infection. In the normal quiescent phase the cervix is closed. During uterine contractions a squeeze-pull effect results in an "in suck" of pathogens into the cervix. During preterm labor the internal cervical os moves cephalad forming a contraction ring. This passive state allows bacteria to be moved up into the lower uterine segment. Note, progressive dilatation of the lower uterine segment, thickening of the myometrial layers in the fundus (active segment), and thinning of these layers in the lower passive segment (50).

the contraction wave moving from the cervix to the fundus. These investigators were concerned that insertion of the endovaginal probe may have caused the observed uterine activity. This is unlikely since a similar type of endometrial movement has been observed using transvesical real-time ultrasonography (64).

CONCLUSION

There is a growing body of evidence to suggest that infection is a significant contributor to poor pregnancy outcome. The current debate focuses on whether infection precedes and causes preterm labor and/or premature rupture of the membranes or whether it is only an associated event. The purpose of this chapter is twofold. *First*, I have attempted to assess our current understanding of genitourinary infections from the point of view of a continuum of risk. There are significant maternal factors that identify a population at greatest risk. This risk begins before pregnancy. We should therefore place particular emphasis on identifying patients at risk before they become pregnant, at a time when intervention may make a difference to the outcome of the future pregnancy. I have next focused on the importance of recognizing the complex problems imposed by asymptomatic infections. It is apparent that we must focus more attention on particular pathogens causing vaginal infection that are different from those causing cystitis and pyelonephritis. There does not appear to be a continuum of risk between the clinical diseases of the genital tract and those of the urinary system, because the pathogens that are associated with preterm birth in these two conditions are different. However since both are associated with premature labor there must be common factors in the pathogenesis.

Finally, I have focused on symptomatic and asymptomatic intrauterine infections. Published reports emphasize the ascending route for both of these infections. The mechanism by which bacteria enter the uterus and establish themselves during pregnancy has not, however, been discussed. I have proposed an active process whereby uterine contractions pull pathogenic bacteria retrogradely into the cervix and lower uterine segment. A second passive mechanism occurs whereby the anatomic changes in the lower uterine segment allow bacteria to move up into the decidual-chorioamniotic space and eventually into the amniotic cavity, initiating the cascade of events leading to preterm delivery.

REFERENCES

1. Bragonier JR, Cushner IM, Hobel CJ. Social and personal factors in the etiology of preterm birth. In: Fuchs F, Stubblefield PG, eds. *Preterm birth: causes, prevention and management*. Ann Arbor: Macmillan, 1984;64–85.
2. Toth A, Lesser ML, Brooks-Toth CW, *et al*. Outcome of subsequent pregnancies following antibiotic therapy after primary or multiple spontaneous abortions. *Surg Gynecol Obstet* 1986;163:243–50.
3. Toth M, Witkin SS, Ledger W, Thaler H. The role of infection in the etiology of preterm birth. *Obstet Gynecol* 1988;71:723–6.
4. McNeeley SG. Treatment of urinary tract infections during pregnancy. *Clin Obstet Gynecol* 1988;31:480–7.
5. Kass EH. Pyelonephritis and bacteriuria: a major problem in preventive medicine. *Ann Intern Med* 1962;56:46–53.
6. Kincaid-Smith P, Bullen M. Bacteriuria in pregnancy. *Lancet* 1965;i:395–9.
7. Romero R, Oyarzon E, Mazor M, *et al*. Meta-analysis of the relationship between asymptomatic bacteriuria and preterm delivery/low birth weight. *Obstet Gynecol* 1989;73:576–81.
8. Savage WE, Hajj SN, Kass EH. Demographic and prognostic characteristics of bacteriuria in pregnancy. *Medicine* 1967;46:385–407.
9. Kunin CM. Epidemiology of bacteriuria and its relation to pyelonephritis. *J Infect Dis* 1969;120:1–12.
10. Duff P. Pyelonephritis in pregnancy. *Clin Obstet Gynecol* 1984;27:17–31.
11. Kass EH. How important is bacteriuria? *Rev Infect Dis* 1982;4:434–37.
12. Waltzer WC. The urinary tract in pregnancy. *J Urol* 1981;125:271–6.
13. Roberts AP, Beard RW. Some factors affecting bacterial invasion of bladder during pregnancy. *Lancet* 1965;1:1133–6.
14. Whalley PJ, Martin FG, Pritchard JA. Sickle cell trait and urinary tract infection during pregnancy. *JAMA* 1964;189:127–30.
15. Turck M, Coffe BS, Petersdorf RG. Bacteriuria of pregnancy: relation to socioeconomic factors. *N Engl J Med* 1962;266:857–60.
16. Minkoff H, Grunebaum AN, Schwarz RH, *et al*. Risk factors for prematurity and premature rupture of membranes: a prospective study of the vaginal flora in pregnancy. *Am J Obstet Gynecol* 1984;150:965–72.
17. Eschenbach DA. Vaginal infection. *Clin Obstet Gynecol* 1983;26:186–202.
18. Gravett MG, Nelson HP, DeRouen T, Critchlow C, Eschenbach DA, Holmes KK. Independent

associations of bacterial vaginosis and chlamydia trachomatis infection with adverse pregnancy outcome. *JAMA* 1986;256:1899–903.

19. Gravett MG, Hummel D, Eschenbach DA, Holmes KK. Preterm labor associated with subclinical amniotic fluid infection and with bacterial vaginosis. *Obstet Gynecol* 1986;67:229–37.

20. Mason PR, Brown IML. Trichomonas in pregnancy. *Lancet* 1980;ii:1025–6.

21. Powell BL, Drutz DJ. Confirmation of corticosterone and progesterone binding activity in candida albicans. *J Infect Dis* 1983;147:359.

22. Mantius T, Krohn MA, Hillier SL, Stamm WE, Holmes KK, Eschenbach D. Relationships of vaginal lactobacillus species, cervical chlamydia trachomatis, and bacterial vaginosis to preterm birth. *Obstet Gynecol* 1988;71:89–95.

23. Hardy PH, Nell EE, Spence MR, Hardy JB, Graham DA, Rosenbaum RC. Prevalence of six sexually transmitted disease agents among pregnant inner-city adolescents and pregnancy outcome. *Lancet* 1984;ii:333–7.

24. Frommell GT, Rothenberg R, Wang SP, et al. Chlamydia infection of mothers and their infants. *J Pediatr* 1979;95:28–32.

25. Handsfield HH, Hodson A, Holmes KK. Neonatal gonococcal infection. I. Orogastric contamination with Neisseria gonorrhoeae. *JAMA* 1973;225:697–701.

26. Lamont RF, Taylor-Robinson D, Newman M, Wigglesworth J, Elder MG. Spontaneous early preterm labor associated with abnormal genital bacterial colonization. *Br J Obstet Gynaecol* 1986;93:804–10.

27. Blanc WA. Amniotic infection syndrome: pathogenesis, morphology and significance in circumnatal mortality. *Clin Obstet Gynecol* 1959;2:705–34.

28. Romero R, Mazor M. Infection and preterm labor. *Clin Obstet Gynecol* 1988;31:553–84.

29. McCormack WM, Rosner B, Lee Y, Muno A, Charles D, Kass EH. Effect on birth weight of erythromycin treatment of pregnant women. *Obstet Gynecol* 1987;69:202–7.

30. Kundsin RB, Driscoll SG, Monson RR, et al. Association of Ureaplasma urealyticum in the placenta with perinatal morbidity and mortality. *N Engl J Med* 1984;310:941–5.

31. Romero R, Mazor M, Oyarzun E, Sirtori M, Wu YK, Hobbins JC. Is genital colonization with Mycoplasma hominis or Ureaplasma urealyticum associated with prematurity low birth weight? *Obstet Gynecol* 1989;73:532–6.

32. Sweet RL. Bacteriuria and pyelonephritis during pregnancy. *Semin Perinatol* 1977;1:25–40.

33. Harris RE, Gilstrap LC. Cystitis during pregnancy: a distant clinical entity. *Obstet Gynecol* 1981;57:578–80.

34. Mimouni F, Miodounik M, Siddigi TA, Berk MA, Wittekind C, Tsang RC. High spontaneous premature labor rate in insulin dependent diabetic pregnant women: an association with poor glycemic control and urogenital infection. *Obstet Gynecol* 1988;72:175–80.

35. Wiederman J, Stone ML, Pataki R. Urinary tract infections and uterine activity. *Am J Obstet Gynecol* 1962;84:290–96.

36. Gilstrap LC, Leveno KJ, Cunningham FG, Whalley PJ, Roark ML. Renal infection and pregnancy outcome. *Am J Obstet Gynecol* 1981;141:709–16.

37. Gibbs RS, Blanco JD, Sinclair PJ, Castaneda YS. Quantitive bacteriology of amniotic fluid from women with clinical intra-amniotics infection at term. *J Infect Dis* 1982;145:1–8.

38. Romero R, Sirtori M, Oyarzun E. Infection and labor. V. Prevalence, microbiology and clinical significance of intra-amniotic infection in women with preterm labor and intact membranes. *Am J Obstet Gynecol* 1989;161:817–24.

39. Bobitt JR, Ledger WJ. Amniotic fluid analysis. Its role in maternal and neonatal infection. *Obstet Gynecol* 1978;51:56–62.

40. Miller JM, Pupkin MJ, Hill GB. Bacterial colonization of amniotic fluid from intact fetal membranes. *Am J Obstet Gynecol* 1980;136:796–804.

41. Wallace RL, Herrick CN. Amniocentesis in the evaluation of premature labor. *Obstet Gynecol* 1981;57:483–6.

42. Bobitt JR, Hayslip CC, Damato JD. Amniotic fluid infection as determined by transabdominal amniocentesis in patients with intact membranes in labor. *Am J Obstet Gynecol* 1981;140:947–52.

43. Wahbeh CJ, Hill GB, Eden RD, Gall SA. Intra-amniotic bacterial colonization in premature labor. *Am J Obstet Gynecol* 1984;148:739–43.

44. Naeye RL, Peters EC. Amniotic fluid infection with intact membranes leading to perinatal death: a prospective study. *Pediatrics* 1978;61:171–7.

45. Hameed C, Tejani N, Verma UL, Archbald F. Silent chorioamnionitis as a cause of preterm labor refractory to tocolytic therapy. *Am J Obstet Gynecol* 1984;149;726–30.

46. Weible DR, Randal HW. Evaluation of amniotic fluid in preterm labor with intact membranes. *J Reprod Med* 1985;30:777–80.
47. Duff P, Kopelman JN. Subclinical intra-amniotic infection in asymptomatic patients with refractory preterm labor. *Obstet Gynecol* 1987;69:756–9.
48. Leigh J, Garite J. Amniocentesis and the management of premature labor. *Obstet Gynecol* 1986;67:500–6.
49. Cederquist LL, Zervovdakis IA, Ewool LC, Litwin SD. The relationship between prematurely ruptured membranes and fetal immunoglobulin production. *Am J Obstet Gynecol* 1979;134:784–8.
50. Keith LG, Bersen GS, Edelman DA, *et al.* On the causation of pelvic inflamatory disease. *Am J Obstet Gynecol* 1984;149:215–24.
51. Friderg J, Fullan N. Attachment of Escherichia coli to human spermatozoa. *Am J Obstet Gynecol* 1983;146:465–7.
52. Galask RP, Varner MW, Petzold CR, Wilbur SL. Bacterial attachment to the chorioamniotic membranes. *Am J Obstet Gynecol* 1984;148:915–28.
53. Naeye RL, Ross S. Coitus and chorioamnionitis: a prospective study. *Early Hum Dev* 1982;6:49–97.
54. Beck JR. How do the spermatozoa enter the uterus? *Am J Obstet* 1874;7:353–91.
55. Heape W. Active suction by the mare uterus during coitus. *The Veterinarian* 1898;71:202–7.
56. Noyes RW, Adams CE, Walton A. Transport of spermatozoa into the uterus of the rabbit. *Fertil Steril* 1958;9:288–99.
57. Hartman CG. How do sperm get into the uterus? *Fertil Steril* 1957;8:403–27.
58. Bickers W. Sperm migration and uterine contractions. *Fertil Steril* 1960;11:286–90.
59. Egli GE, Newton M. The transport of carbon particles in the human female reproductive tract. *Fertil Steril* 1961;12:151–5.
60. Fox CA, Wolff HS, Baker JA. Measurement of intra-vaginal and intrauterine pressures during human coitus by radio-telemetry. *J Reprod Fertil* 1970;22:243–51.
61. Iam JD, Stilson R, Johnson FF, Williams RA, Rice R. Symptoms that precede preterm labor and preterm premature rupture of the membranes. *Am J Obstet Gynecol* 1990;162:486–90.
62. Reynolds SRM. Physiologic relationships in the uterus at term. In: *Physiology of the uterus*, Chapter 37. New York: Hafner Publishing Co, 1965;529–43.
63. de Vries K, Lyons EA, Ballard G, Levi CS, Lindsay DJ. Contractions of the inner third of the myometrium. *Am J Obstet Gynecol* 1990;162:679–82.
64. Birnholz JC. Ultrasonic visualization of endometrial movements. *Fertil Steril* 1984;41:157–8.

DISCUSSION

Dr. Marini: What do you feel about variations in the membranes themselves? Are some more readily penetrated by bacteria than others?

Dr. Hobel: In women with premature rupture of the membranes the force required to rupture the membranes is considerably less than in control women without premature rupture. Thus the membranes are weaker, and I also think that the changes in the lower uterine segment in the presence of infection allow the membranes to rupture more easily. Changes in elastin and collagen occur in preterm labor and these changes presumably affect the membranes. Copper is an important element in collagen synthesis and women with premature rupture of the membranes have been found to have lower copper levels than controls. Thus there may be several reasons why some membranes are more vulnerable than others.

Dr. Saling: Electron microscopic examination of the membranes in cases of amnionitis shows structural damage and in these cases the frequency of premature rupture is as high as 40%, i.e., double the normal frequency of membrane rupture immediately before parturition.

Dr. Marini: A study by Naeye (1) showed that the frequency of sexual intercourse was related to premature delivery. Is this due to mechanical factors increasing the likelihood of bacterial penetration, or is it due to the sperm?

Dr. Hobel: Naeye's study clearly showed that when a condom was used the frequency of premature rupture of the membranes decreased. Thus the sperm appear to play an important role. He also showed that female orgasm increases the likelihood of premature labor.

In relation to obstetric examinations, I feel strongly that no attempt should be made to insert a finger into the cervix. The length of the cervical canal can be readily assessed by examining the posterior part of the cervix.

Dr. Marini: Do you think antibiotic treatment has a place in preventing premature labor?

Dr. Hobel: I have not been impressed by the results of studies in this area. Significant effects have been only borderline. The use of prophylactic antibiotics disturbs the vaginal flora which may itself be harmful. Treating patients when they are symptomatic is appropriate, but efforts should really be directed at preventing bacteria from getting into the lower uterine segment. I am interested in the possibility of preventing colonization by maintaining a low vaginal pH. We also need to know more about uterine motility and how to control it. Some women have retrograde uterine motility.

Dr. Saling: In certain specific cases antibiotic treatment can be helpful. We have observed cases in which C-reactive protein levels were raised in association with symptoms of premature labor, and where treatment with antibiotics resulted in a reduction in uterine activity. The problem is how long to continue treatment for. When we discontinue antibiotic treatment we renew the vaginal flora by application of *Lactobacillus acidophilus* preparations.

Dr. Hobel: We do not do that but it sounds like a good idea. I am sure that it is very important to try to re-establish the normal vaginal flora after treating with antibiotics. I believe in the use of antibiotics in preterm labor because I am convinced there is infection in the lower uterine segment in these cases which is very difficult to diagnose. I am also concerned about the risks to the newborn. I think intrauterine infection plays an important role in confusing our pediatricians about whether there is IRDS or pneumonia.

Dr. Eschenbach: You propose a hypothesis that includes both bacteria and uterine contractions. How would you establish which of these is the more important, or whether a combination of both is required to cause premature rupture of the membranes?

Dr. Hobel: We need to measure uterine activity, monitor vaginal flora, and devise some marker whereby we could study this phenomenon in the human. I was impressed by a paper written in the 1950s in which strips of endometrium obtained from women who had had cesarean sections at term were examined and most showed evidence of infection. I think infection of the uterine cavity is a common phenomenon, but in a small proportion of patients who deliver preterm this may be an overwhelming effect. This suggests that some women have a very low resistance to infection.

Dr. Saling: I think that the general immunologic state of high-risk patients is very important. Papiernik believes that the social state of the patient is a key factor. This is relevant since in people with poor social status the immunological situation is likely to be worse than in people with higher social status, and therefore ascending infection is more likely to have critical consequences.

Dr. Hobel: This makes biological sense. Another factor of interest is the importance of progesterone in stimulating cervical immunoglobulins, which appear to be important in preventing the entry of bacteria. It is possible that women with low progesterone levels may be particularly at risk. I have been impressed by the low frequency of vaginal infections in women who have been given progesterone suppositories because of repeated pregnancy losses at 16 to 20 weeks' gestation. It is possible that vaginal progesterone may prevent colonization with pathogens.

Dr. Marini: Although in most cases of prolonged rupture of the membranes, lung maturation is accelerated, this is not always the case. Do you advocate the use of steroids to enhance lung maturation?

Dr. Hobel: When there is premature labor with very low fetal weight, Dr. Jobe, who does our neonatal pulmonary physiology work, is convinced that corticoids have a beneficial effect on elastin and reduce the risk of bronchopulmonary dysplasia.

Dr. Saling: We give one course of lung maturation therapy in every case of premature rupture of the membranes before 35 weeks' completed gestation. We do not repeat the course if delivery does not occur, because the fact of premature rupture of the membranes itself stimulates lung maturation.

Dr. Eschenbach: Romero has shown a relationship between amniotic fluid infection and respiratory distress in the neonate, but because amniotic fluid infection may be related to low gestational age this is perhaps not surprising. However we have also shown that babies whose placentas contained bacteria had higher rates of IRDS, even when controlling for gestational age. These data suggest that infection in this group may have consequences beyond prematurity alone. Do you have similar data?

Dr. Hobel: There are data to suggest that infection also plays a role in CNS bleeds in preterm infants. Now that we are focusing more on infections during labor, we have an opportunity to help the pediatricians by treating infection. For many years we never gave antibiotics during labor because the pediatricians told us they interfered with their cultures. I think this was a big mistake!

REFERENCE

1. Naeye RL, Ross C. Coitus and chorioamnionitis: a prospective study *Early Hum Dev* 1982;6:91–7.

Perinatology, edited by Erich Saling,
Nestlé Nutrition Workshop Series, Vol. 26,
Nestec, Ltd., Vevey/Raven Press, Ltd.,
New York © 1992.

Laboratory Evidence of Infection Causing Prematurity

David A. Eschenbach

Department of Obstetrics and Gynecology, RH-20, University of Washington, Seattle, Washington 98195, USA

PREMATURITY AND INFECTION

Problem of Prematurity

The rate of premature delivery has remained essentially unchanged over the last 30 years (1). The magnitude of the problem is illustrated by the fact that only 7% of infants are born premature, but these premature infants account for 80% of the perinatal mortality (2). Pregnant women have received the benefit of technologic advances over these 30 years, including antenatal fetal heart rate and ultrasound monitoring, genetic and other prenatal testing, and medication to treat urinary tract infection and premature labor. However, these advances have had a minimal effect upon premature delivery. Fortunately, the perinatal death rate has declined rapidly during this time because premature infants are being optimally cared for by neonatologists.

It is essential to learn more about the pathogenesis of preterm labor. Over half of premature deliveries occur without a known cause. Finding the cause of premature delivery has been hindered by an inability to study many critical sites that could provide clues such as the decidua and placenta until after delivery has occurred. Amniotic fluid obtained before birth can also provide clues to premature delivery. Recently, antepartum amniotic fluid data and postdelivery data from the placenta have indicated that infection can be one factor in preterm delivery. This chapter will examine data relating amniotic fluid and chorioamnion infection to preterm delivery.

Lower Genital Tract Infection

Over the past 30 years, a wide variety of microorganisms recovered from the lower genital tract have been associated with preterm delivery. Higher premature birth rates have been reported among those with, as compared to those without, the following: *Neisseria gonorrhoeae* (3), *Chlamydia trachomatis* (4), group B streptococci

(5), *Ureaplasma urealyticum* (6), *Trichomonas vaginalis* (7), and bacterial vaginosis (8,9). However, none of these microorganisms or infections have been convincingly related in a causal manner to preterm birth. Some microorganisms listed above have not been related to preterm delivery in other investigations and the inconsistency of the findings raises the possibility than confounding factors rather than the microorganisms themselves cause premature labor and birth. Until recently (10), treatment of a specific microorganism has not reduced premature delivery (3) although as presented below, broad spectrum antibiotic therapy aimed at many microorganisms has reduced the rate of preterm delivery. Finally, there has been only limited study (11) of the association between lower and upper genital tract infection. The finding of an association between lower genital tract infection and premature delivery without study of the upper genital tract has always raised questions of whether the microorganisms in question actually gained access to the upper genital tract. The hypothesis that microorganisms cause premature delivery invariably involves a central theme of the ascent of microorganisms from the lower genital tract to the normally sterile upper genital tract. The finding that both lower and upper genital tract infections are related to preterm delivery and, further, the association between lower and upper tract infections, provides convincing data that microorganisms play an active role in some preterm deliveries. In the absence of complete data linking these three points, evidence will be examined for upper genital tract infection in a subset of prematurely delivered pregnancies. It needs to be emphasized that only a proportion of prematurely delivered pregnancies have evidence of infection, perhaps 20–40%, depending upon gestational age.

Antibiotics

A role of microorganisms in prematurity has been inferred from antibiotic trials. In a study conducted from 1963–1965, both nonbacteriuric and bacteriuric women receiving tetracycline in midpregnancy delivered fewer premature liveborn infants than placebo-treated women (12). The antibiotic effect was attributed to the eradication of a tetracycline-sensitive microorganism. Subsequently, 6 weeks of erythromycin therapy in the third trimester was associated with an increased birth weight compared to placebo-treated women (13). Erythromycin therapy was directed at genital mycoplasmas in the latter study, but erythromycin has activity against a wide variety of pathogens associated with prematurity.

More recently, antibiotics have been associated with prolonging pregnancies of women already in preterm labor or with preterm premature membrane rupture. Therapy with ampicillin or erythromycin was given to women in preterm labor with intact membranes. Antibiotic therapy was associated with a statistically significant increase in the time between the onset of preterm labor and delivery in the antibiotic-treated group (30 days) compared to the placebo-treated group (17 days) (14). Patients with premature membrane rupture treated with ampicillin had a significant delay in their delivery compared to placebo-treated patients (15).

TABLE 1. *Relationship of histologic chorioamnionitis to preterm delivery*

Author	Number	Histologic chorioamnionitis		Odds ratio	95% CI
		Preterm	Term		
Russell (16)	7,505	123/659 (19%)	269/6,846 (4%)	5.6[a]	4.4–7.1
Cooperstock *et al.* (17)	18,787	287/1,445 (20%)	817/17,342 (5%)	5.0	4.3–5.8
Guzick & Winn (18)	2,774	80/244 (33%)	253/2,530 (10%)	4.4[b]	3.2–5.9
Fox & Langley (19)	870	16/34 (47%)	186/836 (22%)	3.1	1.5–6.5
Total	29,936	506/2,382 (21%)	1,525/27,554 (5%)	4.6	4.1–5.1

CI, confidence interval.
[a] Birth weight adjusted for gestational age.
[b] Adjusted.

HISTOLOGIC CHORIOAMNIONITIS

Relation to Preterm Delivery

Histologic chorioamnionitis refers to inflammation of the space between the chorion and amnion, often together with inflammation of the umbilical cord and maternal placental floor. The degree of inflammation required for pathologists to make a diagnosis of chorioamnionitis has not been standardized and it undoubtedly varies considerably between studies. Nevertheless, histologic chorioamnionitis has been found more frequently among patients who deliver prematurely than those who deliver at term (16–19) (Table 1). This relationship is consistent in virtually all studies, performed in a variety of populations. The number of cases studied has been large. Histologic chorioamnionitis has been three to five times more common among those who delivered preterm compared to those who delivered at term. The associations between histologic chorioamnionitis and prematurity is strong, consistent, and statistically significant. Small differences of risk are probably related to variations in definitions of chorioamnionitis, in gestational ages, and in prematurity between various populations. With few exceptions, the relationship has not been controlled for potentially confounding factors such as abnormal maternal or pregnancy factors, or labor events such as the length of membrane rupture or labor. However, the strong and consistent relationship between histologic chorioamnionitis and premature delivery is compelling evidence that the two are highly associated.

Inverse Relationship with Degree of Prematurity

Another interesting feature has been the finding that the more premature the delivery, the higher the rate of histologic chorioamnionitis. This striking inverse relationship between gestational age and histologic chorioamnionitis has not been widely examined, but it has been a consistent finding (11,16). The inverse relationship

TABLE 2. *Relationship of chorioamnion infection to preterm delivery*

Author	Chorioamnion infection		Odds ratio	95% CI
	Preterm	Term		
Hillier *et al.* (11)	23/38 (60%)	17/74 (23%)	3.8	1.5–9.9[a]
Kundsen *et al.* (20)				
<1,500 gm	61/196 (31%)	40/312 (13%)	3.1	1.9–4.9[b]
1,500–2,500 gm	48/267 (18%)		1.5	0.9–2.4[b]
Pankuch *et al.* (21)	27/53 (51%)	6/22 (27%)	2.8	0.8–9.4
Svensson *et al.* (22)	8/16 (50%)	33/70 (47%)	1.2	0.3–3.8

CI, confidence interval.
[a] Adjusted using multivariate analysis.
[b] Infection with *U. urealyticum* only.

suggests that either the effect of infection or the fetal-maternal response to infection is not the same throughout pregnancy.

CHORIOAMNIOTIC INFECTION

Relation to Preterm Delivery

Chorioamniotic infection has usually been identified by the recovery of microorganisms from between the chorion and amnion, although in some studies, microorganisms were recovered from the placental floor. The recovery of microorganisms from the placenta does not represent contamination of the placenta by vaginal-cervical microorganisms. Microorganisms common in the vagina, such as lactobacilli, diphtheroids, or *Staphylococcus epidermidis*, are infrequently recovered from the placenta. The presence of microorganisms in the placenta has also been correlated with premature delivery (11,20–22) (Table 2). This finding has been very consistent, except in studies in which normal flora were frequently recovered from term placentas (22) (indicating a problem with specimen contamination). A wide variety of pathogenic bacteria has been isolated from the chorioamnion. *U. urealyticum* has also been a frequent isolate. In one study, *U. urealyticum* accounted for the vast majority of isolates. The relative risk of finding microorganisms in the placenta of preterm compared to term placentas has usually ranged between 1.5 and 4. In studies with a large sample size, the relationship has been statistically significant (11,20). Potentially confounding variables such as the length of rupture of membranes and labor were usually not controlled for in most of these studies. However, the relationship changed little when such factors were controlled by multifactorial analysis (11), indicating limited effect of labor events upon the recovery of microorganisms from this site.

Relation to Histologic Chorioamnionitis

A variety of factors have been invoked as causes of histologic chorioamnionitis, including anoxia and meconium. Recently, the recovery of microorganisms from

TABLE 3. *Relationship of chorioamnion infection to histologic chorioamnionitis*

| | Chorioamnion infection | | | |
	Histologic chorioamnionitis	No histologic chorioamnionitis	Odds ratio	95% CI
Pankuch et al. (21)	18/25 (72%)	6/39 (15%)	14.1	3.6–60
Hillier et al. (11)	21/29 (72%)	14/65 (22%)	7.2	2.7–19[a]
Quinn et al. (23)	10/14 (71%)	8/29 (28%)	6.5	1.3–3.5
Kundsen et al. (20)	32/84 (38%)	21/146 (14%)	3.7	1.8–7.3
Svensson et al. (22)	7/10 (70%)	31/69 (45%)	1.6	0.5–5.0

CI, confidence interval.
[a] Adjusted using multivariate analysis.

between the chorion and amnion has been highly related to histologic chorioamnionitis. The relationship between the two has been remarkably similar. In four studies (11,21–23), microorganisms were recovered from 70% of placentas with histologic chorioamnionitis (Table 3). Histologic chorioamnionitis without the recovery of microorganisms may represent insensitivity of the culture method or membrane inflammation from factors other than infection. The recovery of microorganisms from placentas without histologic chorioamnionitis has ranged more widely, usually from 15–25%. Microorganisms have usually been recovered from placentas with histologic chorioamnionitis two to seven times more often than from placentas without inflammation (11,20–23) (Table 3). The relationship has usually been a statistically significant one, even after controlling for potentially confounding factors (11). Thus, a large proportion of the histologic chorioamnionitis can be explained by the recovery of microorganisms from the chorioamnion.

Inverse Relationship with Degree of Prematurity

Microorganisms are more frequently recovered from the placentas of markedly preterm deliveries than from other preterm or full-term deliveries (11). The inverse relationship between recovery of microorganisms from the placenta and gestational age parallels the inverse relationship between histologic chorioamnionitis and gestational age (11,16).

AMNIOTIC FLUID INFECTION

Relation to Preterm Delivery

Many investigators have reported the recovery of microorganisms from amniotic fluid obtained transabdominally from women in preterm labor. Microorganisms are recovered infrequently from women not in labor. Between 5% and 25% of women in preterm labor have microorganisms in their amniotic fluid (24–32). In a summary

TABLE 4. *Amniotic fluid infection among patients in preterm labor with intact membranes*

Reference	Number	Positive amniotic fluid culture	%
Wallace & Herrick (24)	25	1	4%
Duff & Kopelman (25)	24	1	4%
Skoll *et al.* (26)	127	7	5%
Romero *et al.* (27)	41	4	10%
Hameed *et al.* (28)	37	4	11%
Leigh & Garite (29)	60	7	12%
Gravett *et al.* (30)	54	6	12%
Wahbeh *et al.* (31)	33	4	12%
Bobitt *et al.* (32)	31	8	26%
Total	432	42	10%

of the data in Table 4, 10% of the amniotic fluids obtained from women in preterm labor were culture-positive. The wide range of positive culture results can be attributed, in part, to different culture methods, to whether patients with fever were excluded, and to the gestational age of the pregnancy. As shown for the chorioamnion, a correlation has been noted between positive amniotic fluid cultures and low gestational age (26,27).

Anaerobic bacteria have accounted for about 60% of the isolates from amniotic fluid. Many of the anaerobes are fastidious, which may partly account for the low recovery rate reported from some laboratories. The most common anaerobic bacteria include *Fusobacteria, Bacteroides species*, and *peptostreptococci*. Group B *Streptococci, Gardnerella vaginalis*, and coliforms are the most common facultative isolates. Genital mycoplasmas have also been frequent isolates (27,30).

Relation to Rapid Delivery

The time between amniocentesis and delivery has been 1 day or less for pregnancies in which microorganisms are recovered compared to 25–50 days when microorganisms are not recovered. An exception occurs for the recovery of genital mycoplasmas from amniotic fluid, where there was no relationship between the amniocentesis to delivery interval (30). This finding suggests that delivery occurs quickly when infection of the upper genital tract is severe enough to cause infection of the amniotic fluid.

Relation to Chorioamnion Infection

Unfortunately, there has been no exhaustive study of the relationship of amniotic fluid bacteria to either chorioamnion infection or histologic chorioamnionitis. A consistent relationship between the three would be the key to establishing an ascending

TABLE 5. *Amniotic fluid and serum factor that correlates with amniotic fluid infection*

Amniotic fluid
   Gram stains
      Bacteria
      Polymorphonuclear leukocytes
   Leukocyte esterase
   Endotoxin
   Bacterial metabolic products (gas-liquid chromatography)
   Prostaglandin
   Interleukin
   Leukotrienes
Blood
   Granulocyte esterase
   C-reactive protein
   Leukocyte count

---

route of infection into the upper genital tract along the membrane or decidua. In preliminary studies, we have found that amniotic fluid bacteria are related to the presence of bacteria in the chorioamnion and to histologic chorioamnionitis among patients without membrane rupture. Ascending infection can also occur through ruptured membranes. However, the recovery of microorganisms from amniotic fluid in cases with membrane rupture is difficult to interpret with certainty. With membrane rupture the recovery of bacteria from amniotic fluid could represent either infection or contamination.

Relation to Other Amniotic Fluid Findings

Many amniotic fluid findings indicate that upper genital tract infection exists in a subset of patients who deliver prematurely (Table 5). The clearest data exist for patients with intact membranes where amniotic fluid is relatively uncontaminated from lower genital tract flora. The presence of bacteria, and to a lesser degree polymorphonuclear leukocytes, on Gram-stained amniotic fluid correlates with the recovery of microorganisms (27,33,34). Bacteria or polymorphs in cases with negative cultures could represent culture insensitivity or nonbacterial causes of amniotic fluid inflammatory cells.

Leukocyte esterase is derived, in large part, from polymorphonuclear leukocytes. Leukocyte esterase in amniotic fluid has been correlated with positive amniotic fluid cultures (35). Granulocyte elastase in serum can also be used to indicate infection (36). Neither test has been used among women with idiopathic preterm labor. Raised C-reactive protein levels are common in patients in preterm labor and correlate with an inability to inhibit contractions. C-reactive protein in serum has been correlated with histologic chorioamnionitis in preterm deliveries (37). C-reactive protein was detected in 40% of 40 patients in preterm labor, in none of 10 preterm control patients, and in only one of 12 term control patients (38).

Endotoxin has been detected by a Limulus amebocyte lysate assay in amniotic fluid (27,34) and the presence of endotoxin has been correlated with positive amniotic fluid cultures. Endotoxin was present in amniotic fluid of 69% of culture-positive and only 5% of culture-negative amniotic fluids (34). Endotoxin can cause cellular and endothelial damage and elicit an inflammatory response. Bacterial metabolic products detected by gas-liquid chromatography (GLC) have been correlated with the presence of bacteria in amniotic fluid (33). Metabolic products found by GLC could even represent extra-amniotic infection (39).

One of the postulated pathways of labor involves the production of prostaglandin (40). Prostaglandin levels are higher in the amniotic fluid of women with intra-amniotic infection than of women without infection (38). Prostaglandin levels in amniotic fluid of women with premature rupture of membranes were also higher when the women had a combination of intra-amniotic fluid infection and preterm labor than they were in women with intra-amniotic fluid infection without labor, women in preterm labor without intra-amniotic fluid infection, or women in labor at term (41). These finding suggest that preterm labor involving infection has a different mechanism than labor at term. Prostaglandin may be involved only in preterm labor with intra-amniotic infection. However, the results should be interpreted with caution because membranes were ruptured. Prostaglandins may be produced as a result of decidual or chorioamnion inflammation. In fact, a 30-fold increased level of prostaglandin E was present in the amnion from placentas showing chorioamnionitis compared with placentas without inflammation (42).

Products that result from macrophage stimulation have been found in amniotic fluid, particularly when evidence exists of amniotic fluid infection. Interleukin-1 is a group of polypeptides produced by macrophages, and other cells. Interleukin-1 causes fever and stimulates collagenase and prostaglandin. Decidua stimulated with *Escherichia coli* endotoxin produce interleukin (43). Leukotriene B has been found in increased levels of patients with premature membrane rupture and both labor and intra-amniotic fluid infection (44), and in increased amounts in the amnion of placentas with chorioamnionitis (42).

Relation to Indicators of Neonatal Infection

If both idiopathic respiratory distress syndrome (IRDS) and intra-amniotic fluid infection are related to gestational age, it is not unexpected to find a report relating intra-amniotic fluid infection to IRDS in the infant (27). Intra-amniotic infection was also related to infectious morbidity in the neonate (27). Amniotic fluid infection may be important not only in preterm delivery, but also in enhanced neonatal morbidity. Since both IRDS and neonatal infectious morbidity are highly related to gestational age, it will be important to adjust for gestational age in future studies to determine whether these two events are associated with infection of amniotic fluid/placenta independent of gestational age.

POSSIBLE MECHANISMS

Numerous mechanisms have been proposed by which bacterial infection can cause preterm labor and delivery. Cervical-vaginal bacteria can directly affect the chorioamnion by producing proteases, collagenases, and lipases (45). These enzymes in turn can cause cellular damage to the membrane. Membrane damage could result in membrane rupture or release of prostaglandin and premature labor. Alternatively, bacteria could ascend into the upper genital tract and invade the chorioamnion or decidua and cause an activation of macrophages. Activated macrophages in these tissues would release interleukin, tumor necrosis factor, prostaglandins, and collagenase. These released factors would be expected to affect the membrane directly, or to cause uterine contraction, or both. Products of the bacterial inflammatory response could also cause direct membrane or decidual damage which in turn could release other products that cause uterine contraction.

Complete studies are now required in which these amniotic fluid and serum factors are compared with amniotic fluid and chorioamnion culture results and with histologic chorioamnionitis. Patients with intact membranes should be studied first to avoid possible misinterpretation because of contaminated but not infected specimens. However, current evidence points to infection as a factor in premature delivery of a subset of patients in premature labor or with preterm membrane rupture.

REFERENCES

1. *National Center for Health Statistics: 1951 and 1977. Vol 1. Natality.* U.S. Department of Health, Education and Welfare, Washington D.C.
2. Rush RW, Keirse MJ, Howat P, et al. Contributions of preterm delivery to perinatality mortality. *Br Med J* 1976;2:965–8.
3. Amstey MS, Steadman KT. Symptomatic gonorrhea and pregnancy. *J Am Vener Dis Assoc* 1976;3:14–16.
4. Harrison HR, Alexander ER, Weinstein L, et al. Cervical *Chlamydia trachomatis* and mycoplasmal infection in pregnancy. *JAMA* 1983;250:1721–7.
5. Regan JA, Chao S, James LS. Premature rupture of membranes, preterm delivery and group B streptococcal colonization of mothers. *Am J Obstet Gynecol* 1981;141:184–6.
6. Braun P, Lee Y-H, Klein JO, et al. Birthweight and genital mycoplasmas in pregnancy. *N Engl J Med* 1971;284:167–71.
7. Hardy PH, Hardy JB, Nell EE, et al. Prevalence of six sexually transmitted disease agents among pregnant inner-city adolescents and pregnancy outcome. *Lancet* 1984;ii:333–7.
8. Gravett MG, Nelson HP, DeRouen TA, et al. Independent associations of bacterial vaginosis and *Chlamydia trachomatis* infection with adverse pregnancy outcome. *JAMA* 1986;256:1899–903.
9. Fischbach F, Kolben M, Thurmay R, et al. Genitale Infektionen und Schwangerschaftsverlauf: eine prospektive Studie. *Geburtshilfe Frauenheilkd* 1988;48:469–75.
10. Ryan GM, Abdell RN, McNeeley G, et al. *Chlamydia trachomatis* infection in pregnancy and effect of treatment on outcome. *Am J Obstet Gynecol* 1990;162:34–9.
11. Hillier SH, Martius J, Krohn M, et al. Case-control study of chorioamniotic infection and chorioamnionitis in prematurity. *N Engl J Med* 1988;319:972–8.
12. Elder HA, Santamarina BAG, Smith S, et al. The natural history of asymptomatic bacteriuria during pregnancy: the effect of tetracycline on the clinical course and the outcome of pregnancy. *Am J Obstet Gynecol* 1971;111:441–62.
13. McCormack WM, Rosner B, Lee Y-H, et al. Effect on birth weight of erythromycin treatment of pregnant women. *Obstet Gynecol* 1987;69:202–7.

14. Morales WJ, Angel JL, O'Brien WF, Knuppel RA, Finazzo M. A randomized study of antibiotic therapy in idiopathic preterm labor. *Obstet Gynecol* 1988;72:829–33.
15. Amon E, Lewis SV, Sibai BM, Villar MA, Arheart KL. Ampicillin prophylaxis in preterm premature rupture of the membranes: a prospective randomized study. *Am J Obstet Gynecol* 1988;159:539–43.
16. Russell P. Inflammatory lesions of the human placenta. I. *Am J Diag Gynecol Obstet* 1979;1:127–37.
17. Cooperstock M, England JE, Wolfe RA. Circadian incidence of labor onset hour in preterm birth and chorioamnionitis. *Obstet Gynecol* 1987;70:852–5.
18. Guzick DS, Winn K. The association of chorioamnionitis with preterm delivery. *Obstet Gynecol* 1985;65:11–15.
19. Fox H, Langley FA. Leukocytic infiltration of the placenta and umbilical cord. *Obstet Gynecol* 1971;37:451–8.
20. Kundsen RB, Driscoll SG, Monson RR, *et al*. Association of *Ureaplasma urealyticum* in the placenta with perinatal morbidity and mortality. *N Engl J Med* 1984;310:941–5.
21. Pankuch GA, Appelbaum PC, Lorenz RP, Botti JJ, Schachter J, Naeye RL. Placental microbiology and histology and the pathogenesis of chorioamnionitis. *Obstet Gynecol* 1984;64:802–6.
22. Svensson L, Ingemarsson I, Mardh P-A. Chorioamnionitis and the isolation of microorganisms from the placenta. *Obstet Gynecol* 1986;67:403–9.
23. Quinn PA, Butany J, Taylor J, Hannah W. Chorioamnionitis: Its association with pregnancy outcome and microbial infection. *Am J Obstet Gynecol* 1987;156:379–87.
24. Wallace RL, Herrick CN. Amniocentesis in the evaluation of premature labor. *Obstet Gynecol* 1981;57:483–6.
25. Duff P, Kopelman JN. Subclinical intraamniotic infection in asymptomatic patients with refractory preterm labor. *Obstet Gynecol* 1987;69:756–9.
26. Skoll MA, Moretti ML, Sibai BM. The incidence of positive amniotic fluid cultures in patients in preterm labor with intact membranes. *Am J Obstet Gynecol* 1989;161:813–6.
27. Romero R, Sirtori M, Oyarzun E, *et al*. Infection and labor. V. Prevalence, microbiology, and clinical significance of intraamniotic infection in women with preterm labor and intact membranes. *Am J Obstet Gynecol* 1989;161:817–24.
28. Hameed C, Tejani N, Verma UL, Archbald F. Silent chorioamnionitis as a cause of preterm labor refractory to tocolytic therapy. *Am J Obstet Gynecol* 1984;149:726–30.
29. Leigh J, Garite T. Ammniocentesis and the management of premature labor. *Obstet Gynecol* 1986;67:500–6.
30. Gravett MG, Hummel D, Eschenbach DA, *et al*. Preterm labor associated with subclinical amniotic fluid infection and with bacterial vaginosis. *Obstet Gynecol* 1986;67:229–37.
31. Wahbeh CJ, Hill GB, Eden RD, Gall SA. Intra-amniotic bacterial colonization in premature labor. *Am J Obstet Gynecol* 1984;148:739–43.
32. Bobitt JR, Hayslip CC, Damato JD. Amniotic fluid infection as determined by transabdominal amniocentesis in patients with intact membranes in premature labor. *Am J Obstet Gynecol* 1981;140:947–52.
33. Gravett MG, Eschenbach DA, Spiegel-Brown CA, Holmes KK. Rapid diagnosis of amniotic fluid infection by gas-liquid chromatography. *N Engl J Med* 1982;306:725–8.
34. Romero R, Kadar N, Hobbins JC, Duff GW. Infection and labor: the detection of endotoxin in amniotic fluid. *Am J Obstet Gynecol* 1987;157:815–9.
35. Egley CL, Katz VL, Herbert WNP. Leukocyte esterase: a simple bedside test for the detection of bacterial colonization of amniotic fluid. *Am J Obstet Gynecol* 1988;159:120–2.
36. Fischbach F, Thurmayr R, Kolben M, Graeff H. Possible prediction of neonatal and puerperal infections by intrapartum determination of polymorphonuclear granulocyte elastase levels in maternal blood (letter). *Eur J Clin Microbiol Infect Dis* 1988;7:588–9.
37. Potkul RK, Moawad AH, Ponto KL. The association of subclinical infection with preterm labor: the role of C-reactive protein. *Am J Obstet Gynecol* 1985;153:642–5.
38. Romero R, Emamian M, Quintero R, *et al*. Amniotic fluid prostaglandins levels of and intra-amniotic infections. *Lancet* 1986;i:1380.
39. Iams JD, Clapp DH, Contos DA, Whitehurst R, Ayers LW, O'Shaughnessy RE. Does extra-amniotic infection cause preterm labor? Gas-liquid chromatography studies of amniotic fluid in amnionitis, preterm labor, and normal controls. *Obstet Gynecol* 1987;70:365–8.
40. Schwarze BE, Schultz FM, MacDonald PC, Johnston JM. Initiation of human parturition. IV. Demonstration of phospholipase A-2 in the lysosomes of human fetal membranes. *Am J Obstet Gynecol* 1976;125:1089–92.

41. Romero R, Emamian M, Wan M, Quintero R, Hobbins JC, Mitchell MD. Prostaglandin concentrations in amniotic fluid of women with intra-amniotic infection and preterm labor. *Am J Obstet Gynecol* 1987;157:1461–7.
42. Lopez Bernal A, Hansell DJ, Canete Soler R, Keeling JW, Turnbull AC. Prostaglandins, chorioamnionitis and preterm labour. *Br J Obstet Gynaecol* 1987;94:1156–8.
43. Romero R, Wu YK, Brody DT, Oyarzun E, Duff GW, Durum SK. Human decidua: A source of interleukin-1. *Obstet Gynecol* 1989;73:31–4.
44. Romero R, Quintero R, Emamian M, *et al.* Arachidonate lipoxygenase metabolites in amniotic fluid of women with intra-amniotic infection and preterm labor. *Am J Obstet Gynecol* 1987;157:1454–60.
45. Bejar R, Curbelo V, Davis C, Gluck L. Premature labor. II. Bacterial sources of phospholipase. *Obstet Gynecol* 1981;57:479–82.

DISCUSSION

Dr. Hope: I never believed this business of leaving febrile mothers untreated so that you could culture organisms from the baby. Babies make a very good culture medium but they should not be used as such!

In your list of organisms, with the exception of a few streptococci, you have listed none that we commonly see on our nursery. Maybe there is a difference between our populations, or perhaps our labs are not very good at detection of *Chlamydia, Ureaplasma,* and so on, since I know some places are isolating these organisms more commonly. Of our babies with severe early onset infections, 50% have group B streptococci and the remainder have *Listeria, Haemophilus,* pneumococcus, and a variety of coliforms, none of which feature strongly on your list. If infants are actually dying of pneumonia caused by your unusual organisms, surely we should expect the pathologists to see polymorph infiltration in the lungs, as they do in our culture-positive infants?

Dr. Eschenbach: The most common causes of neonatal bacteremia are group B streptococci and *Escherichia coli.* These account for about 80% of early neonatal bacteremia but are not commonly isolated from the placenta. Thus in these cases bacteremia in the neonate is not related to bacteria in the placenta. If my hypothesis is correct (that the group with evidence of placental infection develop more IRDS and have higher death rates), then either it is a coincidental finding through an indirect mechanism, or it may be that it is much more difficult to isolate these organisms from the neonate than from the adult. Blood cultures on neonates are usually performed on blood samples of less than 1 ml, which are inadequate for these particular bacteremias, where there are usually very few bacteria. Supporting evidence for an indirect hypothesis comes from Gail Cassel's data from Alabama, in which genital mycoplasmas in tracheal aspirates have been related to chronic lung disease in preterm infants.

Dr. Hope: I agree there may well be some indirect explanation. However, if these organisms are causing deaths, the majority of which are occurring in the first days of life, I find it difficult to believe that the pathologists cannot detect them.

Dr. Hobel: We are mainly looking at morbidity today. In the older studies from the 1950s, pathologists commonly made the diagnosis of pneumonia. Today we see few deaths and greater recovery of anaerobic organisms in positive cultures from the mother. The mother is treated, as is the baby, but the pediatrician cannot isolate any organisms and has to decide whether he is dealing with IRDS or some infectious process. However, these babies do not usually die.

Dr. Eschenbach: I am sure that we can successfully treat intrauterine neonatal sepsis in cases where there is maternal febrile illness and evidence of amniotic fluid infection. Although there has been only one randomized study, I think it is clear that neonatal outcome can be improved by treating women with symptomatic infections with antibiotics.

Dr. Roloff: Could you comment on the role of maternal nutrition on infection, including the importance of trace elements such as zinc.

Dr. Eschenbach: The issue of zinc being associated with a bacterial inhibitory factor in the amniotic fluid was documented in the 1970s. It is entirely possible that nutrition is one of the factors explaining the consistent link between low socioeconomic status and preterm delivery. We do not understand the immune mechanisms that may be involved in the high rates of chorioamniotic inflammation and infection in the preterm group, but immunity could also be influenced by nutrition.

Dr. Saling: The most critical group of neonates at risk for infection is without doubt those with premature rupture of the membranes. There is an excellent alternative to antibiotic treatment in these cases that we have been using for many years, and this is to rinse the vagina with dilute iodine solution. This produces a significant reduction in severe infections and we sometimes do it for 2 to 3 weeks prior to delivery. This practice is not well known in the United States.

Dr. Marini: Some recent studies indicate that when mycoplasmas are found very early in tracheal aspirates from preterm babies, the incidence of bronchopulmonary dysplasia is greater. Thus maternal infection may be implicated in chronic neonatal lung disease as well as in preterm delivery.

You showed in most of your cases that there was a rise in PGE_2 and PGI_2. Is indomethacin active in stopping labor?

Dr. Eschenbach: Indomethacin may inhibit labor. Where we consider that amniotic infection is likely to be present we give indomethacin for 48 h with the aim of stabilizing the membranes and inhibiting labor, since we are concerned that delivery may occur before antibiotic treatment has been able to take effect.

Dr. Pollak: You pointed out that if you find a positive amniotic fluid culture the infection is already at a late stage and it may not be possible to intervene successfully. We now treat more and more very small babies for suspected infections but find it difficult to confirm the diagnosis. What is your regimen in trying to select subclinical cases for treatment?

Dr. Eschenbach: I think the simplest way to select patients with possible infections for antibiotic treatment is to study the amniotic fluid for white cells. Ultimately the detection of cytokines may also become a practical way to determine placental infection.

Perinatology, edited by Erich Saling,
Nestlé Nutrition Workshop Series, Vol. 26,
Nestec, Ltd., Vevey/Raven Press, Ltd.,
New York © 1992.

Current Measures to Prevent Late Abortion or Prematurity

Erich Saling

*Department of Obstetrics, Berlin-Neukölln and Institute of Perinatal Medicine,
Free University of Berlin, Mariendorfer Weg 28, D-1000 Berlin 44, Germany*

During the past few years it has been recognized more and more that ascending genital infection is an important factor in the etiology of prematurity. This is confirmed in a number of reports in the literature. Recent reviews have been published by Romero *et al.* (1) and in this volume (see chapters by Eschenbach and Hobel).

In a retrospective study by Schmitz, Riedewald, Schmeling, and myself (unpublished) we have tried to determine the cause of prematurity in 195 cases from our unit with delivery of an infant with a birth weight of less than 2,000 g and gestation less than 37 weeks. The results (Fig. 1) show that in 76% of the cases there was evidence of an infection. This means that there was direct evidence of organisms in the vagina or cervix which are known to be pathogenic or facultative pathogenic, and/or one or more of the following: raised C-reactive protein, IgA against chlamydia (never as a single parameter), leukocytosis, left shift of granulocytes, bacteriuria, abnormal placental histology, or (in several cases) manifest infections in the newborn.

In 29% there was evidence of organisms as well as other signs of infection. In 47% the above-mentioned signs of infection were present but we could not find direct evidence of organisms. In cases where infection was only suspected the incidence of premature rupture of the membranes (PROM) was, as expected, very high, at between 60 and 70%. We think our results show that infection plays a considerable role in causing prematurity.

In principle the course of events is as follows: a functional defect of the cervical barrier and the subsequent ascension of pathogenic organisms leads to local inflammation and prostaglandin release. For example, Bejar and coworkers (2) were able to show that pathogenic organisms like *Bacteroides fragilis* and *Streptococcus viridans* produce phospholipase A_2. This stimulates the arachidonic acid metabolism in the amnion cells and prostaglandin is formed (3). It is also possible that the migration of leukocytes which produces the picture of chorioamnionitis, is also able to induce intrauterine prostaglandin metabolism. According to Romero and coworkers, leukocytes are also able to induce prostaglandin synthesis through the effect of interleukin (4).

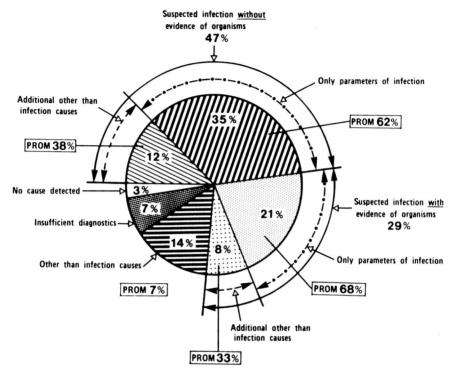

FIG. 1. Causes of premature labor in 195 cases (<37/0 gestational weeks and <2,000 g weight), 1988/89. Data by C. Schmitz, S. Riedewald, S. Schmeling, and E. Saling.

Ascending infections reaching the membranes and decidua can, via the metabolic products of bacteria or local changes due to inflammation, lead to a lessening of the breaking strength of the lower egg pole (5) and, by stimulating prostaglandin synthesis, to premature rupture of the membranes and/or to premature contractions.

At the beginning of the 1990s—and before infection was considered to be so important in the pathogenesis of premature labor—we were able to find the first concrete evidence that a barrier to the ascension of organisms provided much better chances of preventing late abortions or prematurity. To achieve this, since 1981 we have been using the operative early total occlusion of the external os uteri (ETCO), which provides an excellent barrier against the ascension of organisms (6,7). As this measure is only indicated in a small group of high-risk cases with a bad history, we have to search for practicable strategies to prevent dangerous ascending bacteriological infection that can be applied in every pregnancy. On the basis of present knowledge we have elaborated a relatively simple program suitable for daily routine use to prevent late abortions and prematurity in the future and to achieve better overall results (8).

The first important step in our new program is shown in Fig. 2 as Stage I of the routine diagnostic procedures. In the very early stages of pregnancy and then at every subsequent consultation in the antenatal outpatient clinic it is possible—by

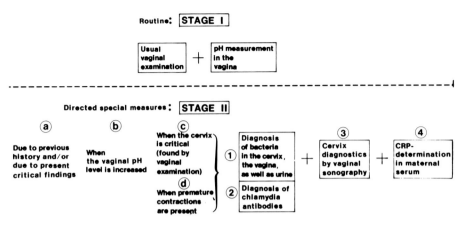

FIG. 2. Diagnostic measures in the prematurity prevention program.

simply measuring the local pH—to find out whether normal, i.e., undisturbed, conditions prevail in the ascending area, particularly in the vagina, so that the ascension of pathogenic organisms can be prevented by the defense mechanisms naturally present—i.e., the vagina must have a relatively high acidity. According to examinations made by our coworker I. M. Kreutzmann, the pH level—measured in the posterior fornix—should be 4.3 or even less (9).

The importance of a normal acidity of the vaginal milieu has been convincingly shown by Ernest and coworkers (10). They found that patients with a mean vaginal pH above 4.5 had a threefold increased risk of premature rupture of the membranes compared with those with a mean pH of 4.5 or lower.

There are three practical ways of measuring the intravaginal pH; all three can be used depending on expected accuracy and on the prevailing situation. The simplest and most precise method is to insert a pH electrode directly into the vagina and to read the pH level using a portable pH meter. The only disadvantage of this method is that the pH electrode must be disinfected after use. This takes about 15 min. The second possibility involves measuring the pH level in a vaginal smear. For this a small but nevertheless adequate amount of vaginal smear must be left on the withdrawn speculum. When the substrate is too small the measurement can be incorrect or even impossible to do. The advantage is that the pH-electrode does not have to be disinfected after use, only cleaned in tap water. The third possibility is to assess the pH level using test paper. This procedure is inexpensive and simple but unfortunately is not so precise as the other two more direct methods.

If the routinely measured pH levels—or other factors—indicate an increased risk, then the measures shown in Stage II (Fig. 2, lower part) should be performed. These are specific diagnostic measures and are necessarily more expensive.

A greater risk is present (on the left of Fig. 2):

a. When indicated by past history, such as previous late abortion or premature birth, and/or when certain critical factors are present in the current pregnancy, such as

poor social status, serious difficulties in professional or family life, multiple pregnancy, uterine anomalies, etc.
b. When the vaginal pH level is increased
c. When the cervix is in a critical state (found by conventional vaginal examination)
d. When premature contractions exist.

When such indications are present, the following diagnostic measures are recommended (on the right of Fig. 2):

1. Bacterial cultures of the cervix and the vagina as well as of the urine
2. Examination of maternal serum for chlamydia antibodies (still controversial)
3. Assessment of the cervix by vaginal sonography
4. Determination of C-reactive protein in maternal serum.

With regard to item 2, it must be said that positive chlamydia IgG and IgA results are naturally not pathognomonic for cervicitis. When there is no direct evidence of a chlamydia infection in the cervix, positive IgA may be the result of a chlamydia infection located in another region. However, when symptoms of threatened premature labor are present and chlamydia antibody tests are positive, it would be careless not to treat because of uncertainty about the precise backgrounds. For this reason we think that antibiotic therapy should be used in such cases.

According to a study made by our coworker E. Hansel (11), cervical assessment by vaginal sonography recommended in point 3 of Stage II appears to be more reliable than the traditional vaginal digital examination alone. If one assumes that a sonographically measured cervical canal length of less than 3 cm can be considered as critical, then it has been shown (Fig. 3) that when the findings on digital examination were normal, with a length of 2 cm or more, nevertheless in almost 20% (left columns) of these cases a shortened cervical canal was measured by vaginal sonography. Such shortening is often due to a three-cornered or sack-shaped hernia-like sacculation of the lower egg pole into the cervical canal in the region of the former inner os uteri. On the other hand in 46% of the cases (Fig. 3, right columns) normal cervical canal lengths were measured by vaginal sonography when short lengths of 1 cm or less had been found by palpation.

C-reactive protein determination can help us in the following ways:

1. It indicates the presence of an overall reaction of the body to a bacteriologically proven ascending infection or urogenital infection and enables an assessment to be made of its degree of severity.
2. Positive C-reactive protein in cases of suspected but unproven infection (negative bacterial cultures) is a helpful piece of evidence that infection is present. In such situations there are risks of premature labor.
3. It allows us to follow the course of the infection and to assess the effect of therapeutic measures.

In an interesting study in 1984, Handwerker and coworkers from New York (12) were able to show that the C-reactive protein levels in the mother have a strong

Length of the portio according to vaginal examination findings

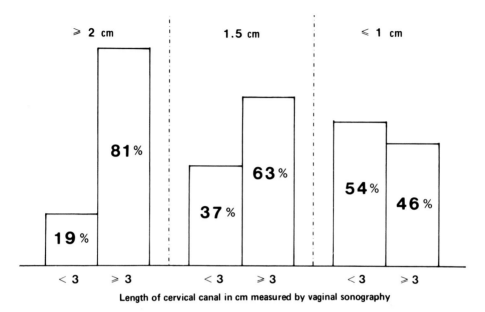

FIG. 3. Relationship between lengths of cervical canal estimated by conventional vaginal examination and lengths measured by vaginal sonography. Data by E. Hansel and E. Saling.

influence on the course of a pregnancy with premature contractions. In a prospective study, the authors found that tocolytic therapy was much more successful in pregnant women who were negative for C-reactive protein. The pregnancy could be maintained in 94% of such cases, but in only 27% of cases that were positive for C-reactive protein. Corresponding birth weights were 2,819 g in the former and only 1,325 g in the latter. These results speak for themselves. We started performing regular C-reactive protein testing 3 years ago and are able to confirm this finding from our clinical observations (13). An increase in C-reactive protein levels can therefore be regarded as an important warning signal. It is, of course, necessary to exclude other infections that lead to increased C-reactive protein levels but that are not critical as far as premature labor is concerned. When determining C-reactive protein concentrations it is important to use a quantitative analytic method with satisfactory precision.

Having gained information from past history and from the various diagnostic methods described, we undertake the following therapeutic measures to reduce the risks of late abortion and prematurity (Table 1).

1. In cases where there have been two or more previous late abortions or premature births we recommend, as initially mentioned, that an ETCO be performed. In this way a complete barrier against ascending infections is achieved. Probably in the

TABLE 1. *Therapeutic measures depending on the risk factors identified in the prematurity prevention program*

	Risk factors	Therapeutic measures
1	≥2 previous late abortions or premature deliveries	Early total operative occlusion of the external *os uteri*
2	Vaginal pH ≥4.4	Acidifying local therapy (*Lactobac. acidoph.*)
3	Evidence of organisms or chlamydia antibodies	Local or systemic antibacterial therapy
4	Critical cervix state and/or premature contractions with increased CRP levels, with no recognizable cause	Systemic broad spectrum antibiotic therapy
5	Critical premature contractions	Tocolysis
6	Critical overall clinical condition	Lung maturity improvement therapy: in urgent cases, betamethason; in less urgent cases, ambroxol

CRP, C-reactive protein.

future we may tend toward a "small total cervical occlusion" which we have recently started performing even after one late abortion or premature birth. This consists of only two to three internal circular stitches completely closing the lower cervical canal, after the glandular epithelium has been removed from this region as far as possible by a rapidly rotating metal brush.

2. Whenever the vaginal pH level is increased above 4.3, therapy using *Lactobacillus acidophilus* preparations should be started to improve the local natural defense mechanisms. This treatment is also indicated at the end of every local or systemic antibacterial therapy. In a study performed by our coworker I. M. Kreutzmann (9), it was clear that vaginal pH levels can be reduced with *Lactobacillus acidophilus* preparations (Fig. 4).

3. If there is evidence of pathogenic organisms in the vagina but the overall situation is not critical, then local therapy can be started, for example in cases with *Candida* or *Trichomonas*. In critical situations when premature contractions have already started and/or the state of the cervix is pathological, or when there is evidence of a chlamydia infection, then we recommend starting systemic antibiotic therapy at once. As far as vaginal acidity is concerned, there are clear connections between positive and negative bacteriological findings and vaginal pH levels. In Kreutzmann's study (9) the mean pH levels measured in the posterior fornix were 4.31 with negative bacteriological findings and 4.91 with positive bacteriological findings.

4. If premature contractions have started and/or the cervix is in a critical state (e.g., the length of the cervical canal is less than 30 mm) in the presence of raised C-reactive protein levels, we recommend admission to hospital and treatment with broad spectrum antibiotics, including agents effective against anaerobes, even if there is no direct evidence of organisms in the vagina, cervix, or urine.

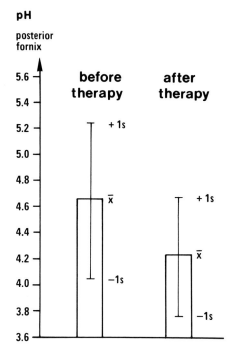

pH

posterior
fornix

FIG. 4. Vaginal pH in cases with premature contractions before and after application of a *Lactobacillus acidophilus* preparation ($\geq$5 days). Data by I. M. Kreutzmann and E. Saling.

5. When critical contractions are present tocolysis should be started for as long as contractions continue and particularly when lung maturation therapy seems necessary. However our view of tocolysis as a whole is that it provides mainly palliative treatment to postpone premature labor temporarily.

6. When premature delivery is imminent, early stimulation of fetal lung maturity must be considered—in acute cases with betamethasone and in less urgent cases with ambroxol.

The first evaluation of this program in our department in conjunction with M. Pluta and C. Schmitz (Fig. 5) shows that it has significantly reduced the incidence of the most critical group of premature infants—namely those with birth weight less than 1,500 g—from 2.0% to 1.3%, a reduction rate of 36%. The delivery of larger premature infants, who are much less endangered, increased concomitantly by 12%. The overall proportion of underweight infants remained unchanged (8.7% and 8.8%). Thus the principal achievement of our program was to postpone premature births until a less dangerous period of gestational age.

Finally I should like to give a short report on our results concerning direct bacteriological access to the lower egg pole, for it is very probable that the decisive process concerned with the onset of premature labor takes place here, as we pointed out at the beginning of the 1980s with the introduction of the ETCO (6,7). In recent years other authors have also produced important supportive evidence for this in

	Before (Jan. 87 – Dec. 88)	After (Jan. 89 – Apr. 90)	Significance
Birth weight in g ╲ Total of infants born	n = 6 519	n = 4 388	
< 1500	n = 132 = **2.0** % ╲ −36%	n = 57 = **1.3** %	p< 0.01
1500 – 2499	n = 436 = **6.7** % +12% ↘	n = 328 = **7.5** %	n. s.
Total < 2500	n = 568 = **8.7** % +0.7% →	n = 385 = **8.8** %	n. s.

FIG. 5. Incidence of low birthweight infants in different groups before and after introduction of prematurity prevention program. Data by M. Pluta, C. Schmitz, and E. Saling.

cases with threatened prematurity, with studies of amniotic fluid taken after transabdominal amniocentesis (14–17). We recently started to achieve direct access to, and have tried to gain bacteriological findings from, the area of the lower egg pole (Fig. 6). A pilot tube, the front part of which is made of silicone, is inserted into the cervical canal. In this pilot tube there is a flexible 1.5 mm plastic catheter (PVC) which fills its lumen. This is introduced a further 2–6 cm according to the state of separation of the membranes from the uterine wall. In this way we can be sure that we have reached the area of the lower egg pole, and that the front end of the inner plastic catheter is in the uterus. Then, using a syringe attached to the outer end of the catheter, 2 ml of sterile 0.9% physiological saline are slowly injected and shortly afterward as much as possible of this solution is aspirated back. When we have recovered more than 0.7 ml (the dead space of the catheter), we can be certain that we have collected fluid that was in contact with the lower egg pole. This fluid undergoes bacteriological examination under anaerobic conditions. A blood culture bottle is also vaccinated and sent off to be examined bacteriologically. A weakness of this lavage method is that it is not yet possible to be certain of preventing some organisms from being carried up the cervical canal. On the other hand, it must be assumed that organisms that have already reached the cervical canal will probably ascend further to the egg pole and can certainly develop pathogenicity there. Organisms from the vagina cannot be transported since the outer os uteri is treated with a disinfectant before catheterization and the device is inserted under visual control directly into the cervical canal.

In the first 25 cases with egg-pole lavage we obtained the following results (with S. Brandt and R. Küchler, Table 2). Positive bacteriologic findings were present in 18 cases. Of these, 13 already had definite symptoms of threatened late abortion or

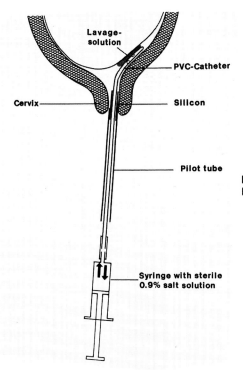

FIG. 6. Diagram showing the lower egg-pole lavage.

premature labor and 5 cases had none. In the groups with symptoms, comprising of 16 patients, 13 cases (81%) had positive cultures with the egg-pole lavage while only 3 cases (19%) had positive bacteriologic findings in the vagina and cervix, using the conventional smear technique.

In the other group at high potential risk, for instance in cases with previous recurrent late abortions, organisms were found at the lower egg pole in five out of nine cases, but only one case was positive using the conventional swab technique.

From these results—drawn from a small group—it is not possible to say with certainty whether the cultured organisms were alone responsible for the critical clinical situation. We are just beginning this study and it needs time for further development. There is at present no evidence that this new technique has any serious side effects. Slight contact bleeding which was observed in 3 out of 25 cases immediately after the procedure ceased within the first 2 h and was seen only in one case examined 3 to 5 h after lavage. No serious contractions or rupture of the membranes occurred within 48 h, so no such events could be connected with the procedure. The possibility that bacteria might be introduced into the uterus by the catheterization procedure cannot be overlooked, but in principle there are no essential differences between this technique and the manipulation required for the conventional cervical smear technique which has been common for a long time, for instance for the diagnosis of *Chlamydia*.

TABLE 2. *First results of lower egg-pole lavage in cases of potential high risk or in cases with definite symptoms of threatened late abortion or prematurity[a]*

Symptoms of threatened late abortion or prematurity	Total	Evidence of organisms	Organisms plus CRP >1.0 mg/dl	Evidence of pathogenic organisms in vaginal or cervical smear by conventional swab technique
None, but potential high risk (e.g., recurrent abortion); Gestational age 9/5–26/1	n = 9	n = 5 (56%)	n = 0	n = 1 (11%)
Definite; Gestational age 22/3–34/6	n = 16	n = 13 (81%)	n = 9 (56%)	n = 3 (19%)
All cases	n = 25	n = 18 (72%)	n = 9 (36%)	n = 4 (16%)

[a] In the middle line group of patients several cases are included in which no bacterias were found in the vagina or in the cervix using the conventional swab technique in a previous examination. Therefore, the search has been continued using egg-pole lavage and consequently the number of cases—only 3 (19%) is relatively low.
CRP, C-reactive protein.
Data by S. Brandt, R. Küchler, and E. Saling.

Concerning our whole prematurity prevention program I am fully aware of gaps in our knowledge, and there are of course many more questions remaining to be answered. Nevertheless this work shows that positive results are achievable. We find ourselves in a very typical situation of intuitive clinical management which frustrates the theorist and provokes the dogmatist, because of the lack of a prospective study, but which gives well-grounded hope to the practical obstetrician.

REFERENCES

1. Romero R, *et al.* Infection in the pathogenesis of preterm labor. *Semin Perinatol* 1988;12:4.
2. Bejar R, Curbello V, Davis C, Gluck L. Premature labor and bacterial sources of phospholipase. *Obstet Gynecol* 1981;57:473.
3. Bennett PR, Rose MP, Myatt L, Elder MG. Preterm labor stimulation of arachidonic acid metabolism in human amnion cells by bacterial products. *Am J Obstet Gynecol* 1987;156:649.
4. Romero R, Mitchell M, Duram S. A possible mechanism for premature labor in gram negative maternal infection; a monocyte product stimulates prostaglandin release by the amnion. *32nd Annual Meeting Society of Gynecological Investigation*, 1985; [Abstract] 219.
5. Sbarra AJ, Thomas GB, Cetrulo CL, Shakr C, Chaudbury A, Paul B. Effect of bacterial growth on the bursting pressure of fetal membranes in vitro. *Obstet Gynecol* 1987;70:107.
6. Saling E. Der frühe totale Muttermundverschluß zur Vermeidung habitueller Aborte und Frühgeburten. *Z Geburtshilfe Perinatol* 1981;185:259.
7. Saling E. Early total operative occlusion of the cervix for prevention of recurrent late abortions. Presented at the *9th Annual Meeting of the Society of Perinatal Obstetricians*, Feb. 1989; New Orleans, LA, USA.
8. Saling E. Zusätzliche aktuelle Maßnahmen zur Vermeidung von Spätaborten und Frühgeburten. Vortrag beim 14. Deutschen Kongreß für Perinatale Medizin, Berlin 4. Oct. 1989. In: Dudenhausen JW, Saling E, eds. *Perinatale Medizin*, Vol XIII. Stuttgart: Thieme, 1990.

9. Kreutzmann IM, Riedewald S, Saling E. Vaginale pH-Werte bei normaler und pathologischer Schwangerschaft. In: Dudenhausen JW, Saling E, eds. *Perinatale Medizin*, Vol XIII. Stuttgart: Thieme, 1990.
10. Ernest JM, Meis PJ, Moore ML, Swain M. Vaginal pH: a marker of preterm premature rupture of the membranes. *Obstet Gynecol* 1989;74:734.
11. Hansel E. Doctoral thesis at the Free University of Berlin, 1991.
12. Handwerker SM, Tejani NA, Verma UL, Archbald F. Correlation of maternal serum C-reactive protein with outcome of tocolysis. *Obstet Gynecol* 1984;63:220.
13. Bell U, Kynast G, Saling E. Die Bedeutung der CRP-Bestimmung für die Diagnostik bei aszendierenden Infektionen und drohender Frühgeburt. Doctoral thesis at the Free University of Berlin. [In preparation.]
14. Skoll MA, Moretti ML, Sibai BM. The incidence of positive amniotic fluid cultures in patients in preterm labor with intact membranes. *Am J Obstet Gynecol* 1989;161:813–6.
15. Romero R, Sirtori M, Oyarzun E, *et al*. Infection and labor V. Prevalence, microbiology, and clinical significance of intraamniotic infection in women with preterm labor and intact membranes. *Am J Obstet Gynecol* 1989;16:817–24.
16. Leigh J, Garite T. Amniocentesis and the management of premature labor. *Obstet Gynecol* 1986;67:500–6.
17. Gravett MG, Hummel D, Eschenbach DA *et al*. Preterm labor associated with subclinical amniotic fluid infection and with bacterial vaginosis. *Obstet Gynecol* 1986;67:229–37.

DISCUSSION

Dr. Eschenbach: The raised pH is probably related to the increased numbers of organisms found in patients with bacterial vaginosis. There have been at least three studies in the United States relating bacterial vaginosis to preterm delivery, which would be entirely consistent with your findings. The issue of contamination of cervical samples with lower genital tract bacteria is particularly important in patients with pelvic inflammatory disease. Are the organisms contaminants or were they really in the uterine cavity? You might consider doing a Gram stain of the lower vagina to look for the presence of bacterial vaginosis, when organisms are present in concentrations a thousand times higher than in women without vaginosis.

Dr. Saling: I agree. We would do this in cases where bacterial vaginosis is suspected. But in many cases the vaginal milieu appears to be normal and in such cases, or when you have negative results with the swab technique, you can then try egg-pole lavage. This should only be done as a further step.

Dr. Hoyme: Several studies have shown that IgA persists for months. Did you follow up your patients who had had chlamydia IgA serology?

Dr. Saling: No, we did not. But as clinicians we have to treat such cases in critical situations. If we find a high IgA with no other explanation we give the patient erythromycin for a relatively long period, 2 to 3 weeks or longer if necessary. We don't know exactly whether we are on the right track, but if we have contractions there is a critical cervical state, so even if there is no other evidence of infection we think it justified to treat in this way.

Dr. Marini: Your rate of 2% of very low birth weight in untreated cases is quite high by Western European standards. We have a lower rate in Italy. Is this related to the immigrant population in Berlin?

Dr. Saling: Because we are a well-known center we get transfers of high-risk patients from other departments and from practitioners. There is also a relatively high proportion of foreigners in our population.

Dr. Marini: In relation to chlamydia, you said that you measure specific IgA and IgG. Why not IgM? Would not this be of interest too?

Dr. Küchler: Chlamydial infection of the vagina and cervix is considered to be a local infection, so the IgM response is not a very important one, whereas the IgA response is highly reliable.

Dr. Eschenbach: However, preterm birth is more highly related to chlamydial IgM than IgG serum antibody.

Dr. Hobel: Closure of the cervix is an intriguing approach to the prevention of ascending infection. Could you tell us when is the best time to perform the procedure and what exactly it is that you do?

Dr. Saling: We usually perform total cervical occlusion as an early preventive measure, that is at about 12 weeks of gestational age and before there is any detectable anatomic change of the cervix. If the patient is transferred later than this we may carry out a "late" occlusion which is better than nothing, but not as good as an early occlusion.

Under anesthesia we remove the epithelium with a rotating wire brush to a radius of about 10 mm from the external os. The epithelium must be removed because otherwise the adapted tissue will not heal. We carry out the same procedure in the cervical canal to a depth of about 15 mm. We then perform two to three circular sutures in the cervix so that the cervical canal becomes totally closed. Afterward the external os is stitched twice with two transverse rows of sutures.

At first we kept these patients in hospital, but now we allow them home, with intensive prenatal follow-up care. We admit them again 2 weeks before term and open the scar under local anesthesia, which is not difficult. The cesarean rate in the group is only about 15%. Three to four weeks after delivery we check the cervix in the clinic. In most cases the portio is in similar condition to its preoperative state.

In our patient series we now achieve a live infant in about 80% of cases whereas this same patient group untreated has only about a 17% chance of a surviving infant. The closure of the cervical canal prevents ascending infection and the good results are convincing proof that most late abortions or very early premature births are caused by ascending infection.

Dr. Marini: How do you introduce lactobacilli?

Dr. Saling: This is easy because preparations are available. The patient inserts a *Lactobacillus acidophilus* vaginal suppository, obtained from a pharmacy, each evening on going to bed, depending on the pH level. If the effect is not sufficient, two should be inserted, one in the morning and one in the evening. When vaginal pH values return to normal (4.3 or less) the intervals of application can be prolonged to 2 to 3 days.

Perinatology, edited by Erich Saling,
Nestlé Nutrition Workshop Series, Vol. 26,
Nestec, Ltd., Vevey/Raven Press, Ltd.,
New York © 1992.

The Clinical Value of Extracorporeal Membrane Oxygenation

Dietrich W. Roloff

Newborn Services and Pediatric Pulmonary Medicine, Department of Pediatrics, University of Michigan, Ann Arbor, Michigan 48109, USA

BACKGROUND

Clinical perinatology to a large extent concerns itself with the maintenance of normal respiratory gas exchange for fetus and neonate via placenta and lungs. Disturbances in the function of these organs account for most perinatal morbidity and mortality.

Thus, the progress in the care of infants with respiratory failure is widely identified with advances in mechanical ventilation (although one should certainly acknowledge the vastly improved nutritional care of sick newborns as well). However, those who treat these infants realized that mechanical ventilation not only has its limits of efficacy, but that it may actually contribute to further pathology by its principal mechanisms, namely oxygen and pressure. Moreover, since most neonatal pulmonary failure is limited in duration, respirator treatment is not so much therapy but rather support of the patient until the pathophysiological process has run its course. Therefore, it was an early dream of clinicians that total support by means of cardiopulmonary bypass would afford a more logical and, therefore, more effective mode of intervention. Early attempts by Saling, and White *et al.* in the 1960s failed because their concepts were ahead of available technology. The alternative strategy of replacing surfactant when its deficiency is the cause of neonatal respiratory failure is being addressed by Prof. Fujiwara elsewhere in this volume.

We should emphasize here that the basic principle of these strategies is the reversibility of the underlying lung disease whereby the patient is supported during recovery. Now that extracorporeal membrane oxygenation (ECMO) has indeed become a reality we may well ask if it has fulfilled these dreams. Does it allow the obstetrician the deliberate delivery of a premature infant because a continued pregnancy will be detrimental to the fetus? Will the pediatrician be able to use it in lieu of the unphysiological parameters of mechanical ventilators? Has it improved survival — has it improved "quality" survival?

TECHNIQUE

ECMO for the purpose of this presentation describes the veno-arterial cardio-pulmonary bypass in newborns above 35 weeks' gestational age. Thus, we can state that at present the answer to the original question, namely, the support of prematures in the sense of replacing the placenta, has not yet been found.

The ECMO circuit drains venous blood from the right ventricle by gravity; a roller pump drives the blood through a membrane lung and a warmer into the patient's aortic arch (1). The patient's blood is anticoagulated with heparin. The vascular connections require the entry into and ligation of the carotid artery and the jugular vein. These technical necessities present risks and are indeed major reasons for considering ECMO as hazardous. However, as with technical problems in general, they are being addressed— single cannula/dual lumen veno-venous circuits have already been successfully used in some 50 cases at our institution, and we are about to introduce heparin-coated circuits.

A typical patient will require 4–5 days of bypass during which time he remains on low ventilator settings and will be awake with mild sedation. Antibiotics and intravenous nutrition are given, and blood and platelets are replaced. The administration of pressors is rarely necessary.

To accomplish all of this, a well-trained ECMO team must be available at short notice because the infants are extremely unstable and hypoxic, indeed moribund, i.e., with an 80% chance of dying, when they meet criteria for ECMO. Typically, oxygen tension values are below 45 torr, whereas inspiratory ventilator pressures exceed 40 cm H_2O. An experienced team will have the circuit primed, the patient cannulated, and bypass flow established within about 90 min of the decision to proceed. Immediately afterward, the clinical value of ECMO becomes apparent: the patient will be hemodynamically stable and well-oxygenated while pressor drips have been discontinued and mechanical ventilation parameters reduced to nominal settings. The continuous presence at the bedside of specifically trained ECMO technicians assures attention to numerous details; especially important is the control of systemic heparinization by keeping the activated clotting time within narrow limits. Complications arising from the circuit include failure of the membrane lung, rupture of the tubing, and clot formation. Patient-related events are seizures, hypertension, and hemorrhages.

CLINICAL USE AND RESULTS

ECMO is now being performed at over 60 hospitals in at least six countries. A professional group, the Extracorporeal Life Support Organization (ELSO), was founded in 1989, and two conferences on ECMO are held each year. A registry of all cases performed at participating centers is maintained by ELSO and contains information on 3,715 cases entered by April 1990, of which 83% survived. Just over 1,000 neonatal ECMO procedures were done in each of the last 2 years. This leveling off is interesting because at this rate there was about one ECMO case per 3,500 newborns in the United States each year, a ratio that had been calculated as the approximate need for ECMO. It remains to be seen if saturation has occurred.

Who are these moribund neonates we expect to benefit from ECMO? As noted above, all are in severe respiratory failure as determined by measures of hypoxemia, such as the alveolar-arterial oxygen gradient over 600 torr or an oxygenation index approaching 40. Most ECMO centers have arrived at their criteria in this range by retrospective analysis of cases during the period preceding the introduction of ECMO for the purpose of defining values from which 80% mortality can be defined. When attempting to determine the "correct" cutoff point, one has to deal with the fundamental problem of deciding if it is preferable to expose any infants who would have survived without ECMO to its procedural risk or if it is acceptable to have anyone die on continued conventional support who would have lived because ECMO was used. Thus, we have calculated that about 27 carotid arteries not ligated correspond to one prevented infant death when using fairly strict criteria and current complication rates.

The registry data identify the various causes of respiratory failure in neonates and their success rates with ECMO. The most common indications (about half) are meconium aspiration syndrome and persistent pulmonary hypertension. This has also the best survival rate of up to 95%. Near-term and term infants with the clinical diagnosis of respiratory distress syndrome (RDS) come next (15%), with a survival of 83%. Increasingly, the lower range of acceptable degrees of prematurity for ECMO are being probed— several 33- to 34-week infants have been successfully treated without any undue complications. When it comes to infants with the diagnosis of pneumonia, mostly due to group B streptococcal sepsis (12%), the failures become more common (76% survival). Various other reasons to employ ECMO include recurrent pneumothorax or cardiac disease.

An indication apart is the infant with congenital diaphragmatic hernia (CDH). Few conditions have resisted the improvements in neonatal intensive care and surgery as has CDH. With the advent of ECMO, an additional means of support, both pre- and postoperatively has become available. The increasing proportion of prenatally sonographically diagnosed cases of CDH has stimulated the discussion of whether or not it should be recommended that all these infants be born at hospitals with ECMO availability. Survival is 62%. Fascinating results of intrauterine surgical repair of CDH by Dr. Harrison's team in San Francisco are presented by Dr. Golbus in this volume.

Follow-up examinations identify about 15% neurologically impaired survivors in whom it is often difficult to differentiate the effects of pre-ECMO events from that of the procedure itself (2). We have found a 5% incidence of right-sided cerebral infarcts; others have not.

COST

Having described the resources needed one should ask about the cost of ECMO. How expensive is it and is it cost-effective? As to the relative cost of it, each day

TABLE 1. *Costs and outcome of neonatal ECMO*

| | | Days | | | | Abnormal at discharge | |
Group	n	Vent.	NICU	Hospital	US$	Respiratory %	Neurological %
A	18	11	18	26	57,600	28	22
B	5	13	21	34	67,058	40	80
C	12	9	19	27	53,687	0	8
D	20	9	14	24	52,076	15	20

Group A: Moderate respiratory failure, ECMO, criteria not met, conventional treatment.
Group B: Severe respiratory failure, no ECMO.
Group C: Severe respiratory failure, randomized to early ECMO.
Group D: Severe respiratory failure, randomized to late ECMO.

on ECMO costs about as much again as one intensive care day. That is, an ECMO patient will cost double to triple the price of an NICU patient not on ECMO. In absolute terms the daily NICU charge in the United States now is about $1,500. Another way to express the impact of ECMO is the comparison to other treatments such as bone marrow transplant, fetal surgery, or surgery for congenital heart disease.

We have attempted to determine the cost-effectiveness of ECMO and compared hospital charges, ventilator days, and hospital stay in three groups of infants: early ECMO, late ECMO, and no ECMO (Tables 1 and 2). We found that the ECMO patients had about the same hospital bills, primarily because they had fewer days in the intensive care unit. We concluded that the improved ECMO survival was achieved without increasing hospital utilization, or morbidity. A comment on the inconsistency in applying cost-benefit analysis and setting priorities in health care might be the fact that in the United States about the same amount of money is spent for circumcisions as for ECMO. One can also compute that ECMO lowers the infant mortality by about 2%.

TABLE 2. *Follow-up examination at one year*

| | | | Abnormalities | |
| | | Normal | Respiratory | Neurological |
Group	n	%	%	%
A	16	50	38	12
B	5	20	80	40
C	12	67	33	0
D	20	65	30	5

EFFICACY

We are often asked about controlled studies demonstrating efficacy. Two such studies have been done. Both used an adaptive study design. In such a study, the outcome of a patient randomized to receive either ECMO or conventional treatment will increase the chance of the next patient being assigned to the more promising treatment. As a consequence, our own study (3) contained only one control patient (who died), whereas all 11 ECMO patients lived. A second similar but larger and statistically more sophisticated study in Boston (4) saw four of ten control infants die and all nine ECMO babies survive— randomization was then stopped and ECMO offered to all who qualified, with 19 of the next 20 surviving.

These studies have generated intense debate about research methodology and ethics (5)—four editorials (6–9) in one journal alone, as well as an article in the *Boston Globe* are testimony to this controversy. Thus, in addition to all its other contributions, ECMO has been a paradigm of introducing new technology into patient care.

CONCLUSIONS

In summarizing the experience with ECMO so far the critical questions to be asked are:

1. *Is extracorporeal membrane oxygenation needed?*

Any time a method improves survival as drastically as ECMO has, one should consider that the conventional "optimal" therapy was not really optional. Improved understanding of ventilator management, e.g., high-frequency ventilation (10) or the approach of avoiding hyperventilation advocated by Wung et al. (11), and maybe surfactant and improved peripartum management as prevention, may give the answer that ECMO will still be needed but possibly not as much.

2. *Is ECMO as described here the best method?*

Quite likely not. At the very least it will be simplified and automated. Other circuits will be introduced—veno-venous as already mentioned, or maybe even arterio-venous, as proposed by S. Schmidt. Also further work is needed to compare different physiological strategies such as removing CO_2 rather than supplying oxygen.

Against these critical questions I assess the current role of extracorporeal membrane oxygenation as that:

1. It works.
2. It is acceptably safe.
3. It is affordable.
4. Long-term outcomes are satisfactory.

REFERENCES

1. Bartlett RH, Gazzaniga AB, Toomasian J, Coran AG, Roloff D, Rucker R. Extracorporeal membrane oxygenation (ECMO) in neonatal respiratory failure. 100 cases. *Ann Surg* 1986;204:236–45.
2. Glass P, Miller M, Short B. Morbidity for survivors of extracorporeal membrane oxygenation: neurodevelopmental outcome at one year of age. *Pediatrics* 1989;83:72–8.
3. Bartlett RH, Roloff DW, Cornell RG, Andrews AF, Dillon PW, Zwischenberger JB. Extracorporeal circulation in neonatal respiratory failure: a prospective randomized study. *Pediatrics* 1985;76: 479–87.
4. O'Rourke PP, Crone RK, Vacanti JP, *et al.* Extracorporeal membrane oxygenation and conventional medical therapy in neonates with persistent pulmonary hypertension of the newborn: a prospective randomized study. *Pediatrics* 1989;84:957–63.
5. Lantos JD, Frader J. Extracorporeal membrane oxygenation and the ethics of clinical research in pediatrics. *N Engl J Med* 1990;323:409–13.
6. Ware JH, Epstein MF. Extracorporeal circulation in neonatal respiratory failure; a prospective randomized study. *Pediatrics* 1985;76:849–51.
7. Nelson NM. Of hummingbirds, extracorporeal membrane oxygenation, and IBM. *Pediatrics* 1990;85:374–6.
8. Chalmers TC. A belated randomized trial. *Pediatrics* 1990;85:366–9.
9. Meinert CL. Extracorporeal membrane oxygenation trials. *Pediatrics* 1990;85:365–6.
10. Carter JM, Gerstmann DR, Clark RH, *et al.* High frequency oscillatory ventilation and extracorporeal membrane oxygenation for the treatment of acute neonatal respiratory failure. *Pediatrics* 1990;85: 159–64.
11. Wung JT, James LS, Kilchevsky E, James E. Management of infants with severe respiratory failure and persistence of the fetal circulation, without hyperventilation. *Pediatrics* 1985;76:488–94.

DISCUSSION

Dr. Johnson: What prevents you from using this system for more premature infants?

Dr. Roloff: The main reason is the risk of intraventricular hemorrhage. This may be the result of alterations in the cerebral blood flow, not just from ligation of the carotid artery but also from changed patterns of perfusion. The pump provides nonpulsatile blood flow and different organs vary in their tolerance to nonpulsatile flow. The age for the procedure has, however, gradually edged downward, and we have now treated a few patients of 32 to 34 weeks without causing intraventricular hemorrhage. We check all patients sonographically and exclude any with more than a grade I IVH.

Dr. Saling: When we started this method in a very primitive way in the 1960s there was a high rate of hemolysis. Do you find this with modern machines as well? And what is the infection risk?

Dr. Roloff: The use of membrane rather than bubble oxygenators is one of the reasons why red cells are now less damaged mechanically. We test daily for raised serum hemoglobin as a means of surveillance. With heparinization and flow rates of around 120 ml/kg·min, one does not see excessive mechanical hemolysis. The infection risk is surprisingly low, with significant infections occurring in only about 1–2%.

Dr. Marini: I have heard that renal complications are frequent with ECMO. Is this true?

Dr. Roloff: A degree of renal failure is perhaps not so much a complication as an inevitability in ECMO. It relates to the nonpulsatile blood flow, which the kidney is intolerant to. Urine output decreases, and fluid shifts occur, with water moving into the tissues, including the lungs. A weight gain of 500–1,000 g may occur on the first 2 days, requiring the use of a hemofilter. This renal failure is reversible. We believe that the introduction of a pulsatile flow system would make the pump and circuitry more complex, with only limited benefit.

Dr. Hobel: It sounds as if some of the renal problems may be the result of impaired release of atrial natriuretic factor (ANF) from the atrium. Has anyone considered giving ANF to improve urine production?

Dr. Roloff: Many people are talking about this and it is a logical thing to consider, but I am not aware of any studies. Hypertension after ECMO is not uncommon, with extremely high renin levels in some patients.

Dr. Hope: One reason for not wishing to embark on a new technique such as this is lack of resources, and I noted the acknowledgment of a huge list of people involved in your first studies of technique. What worries me is that, having started off as you did by treating patients whom you assumed would have an 80% mortality on conventional treatment, ECMO has now become available in so many centers in the USA that more patients are now being treated than would be expected to die with conventional treatment. It is also worth recalling that the assumption that 80% of treated babies would have died on conventional treatment is an *assumption*, not a fact. We still don't have a suitable trial. The Boston trial was extraordinarily designed. A rather more secure, if maybe less sophisticated, statistical design is required.

Dr. Roloff: Of course what was true 2 years or so ago may no longer be true. But we had to arrive at our criteria retrospectively to make decisions from blood gases, ventilator settings, and oxygen use in order to determine our cutoff points. The dilemma is always the same: do you wish to prevent even one patient getting ECMO who did not need it? Or do you wish to prevent even one patient dying who would have lived because of ECMO? We have calculated that in our center 27 carotid arteries not violated are equivalent to one dead baby.

The question of whether our "conventional" treatment was not optimal deserves serious consideration. One important factor may be the large variance in meconium aspiration. Colleagues from several European countries have told me that they hardly remember when they last saw a case of severe meconium aspiration in their own center. So there may be problems more applicable to our particular population than to others. Any time that a new treatment works in 90% of the patients who had a 80% mortality before, you wonder whether your mortality figures were wrong or your "conventional" treatment was wrong. Consider that ECMO may work primarily because it allows conventional treatment to be stopped. Whatever the factors, at the time of decision for ECMO all these patients are severely hypoxic.

Dr. Pollak: With persistent fetal circulation, do you use ECMO from the start or only after the failure of conventional therapy?

Dr. Roloff: Conventional therapy is hard to standardize. Some consider that tolazoline is essential, others that it is detrimental. We always try vasoactive agents and hyperventilation first before moving to ECMO.

Dr. Pollak: Along the lines of what you were saying before about differences in treatment populations, in our own institution, where we use hyperventilation therapy alone, we do not see severe persistent fetal circulation syndrome that is unresponsive to conventional treatment.

Dr. Roloff: Of course there are others who have suggested that hyperventilation treatment has a higher morbidity and mortality. One needs to separate hospital statistics from population statistics. Much depends on how primary hospitals cover deliveries, especially of post-dates pregnancies. Many of our patients with meconium aspiration syndrome are from post-dates deliveries.

Dr. Pollak: You showed a high rate of neurological abnormality of about 40% in some of your infants with severe respiratory failure. What type of cases were these?

Dr. Roloff: Many had birth asphyxia with hypoperfusion as well as hypoxia. The group as a whole had fairly good Apgar scores, but infants with particularly poor pre-ECMO courses are at highest risk. Infants with persistent fetal circulation who were in fairly good condition initially may have extremely low oxygen saturations but still do well afterward, whereas infants with initial hypoperfusion do much more poorly.

Perinatology, edited by Erich Saling,
Nestlé Nutrition Workshop Series, Vol. 26,
Nestec, Ltd., Vevey/Raven Press, Ltd.,
New York © 1992.

Clinical Value of Magnetic Resonance and Near-Infrared Spectroscopy in Neonates

Peter Hope, Kevin Ives, and James Moorcraft

Department of Paediatrics, John Radcliffe Hospital, Oxford OX3 9DU, England

There is no doubt that cerebral ultrasound has proved an extremely useful technique for the neonatologist, who is increasingly concerned not only with reducing perinatal mortality but also with improving the quality of neonatal survival. Over the last decade, we have learned a great deal about the pathogenesis, natural history, and prognosis of periventricular hemorrhage in preterm infants, which is ideally demonstrated by ultrasound. However, ultrasound is less satisfactory for the early detection of cerebral hypoxic-ischemic lesions which are now recognized as a major cause of severe neurodevelopmental problems in preterm survivors (1). The motivation to explore other technologies for investigating the newborn brain, such as magnetic resonance spectroscopy (MRS) and near-infrared spectroscopy (NIRS) stems from the inadequacy of conventional techniques for studying cerebral ischemic lesions. This applies not only to preterm infants, but also to full-term infants who suffer hypoxic-ischemic encephalopathy following severe birth asphyxia, because these infants also contribute considerably to the toll of perinatally acquired handicap in the community.

PHOSPHORUS-31 MAGNETIC RESONANCE SPECTROSCOPY (^{31}P MRS)

MRS has been used as a nondestructive technique of biochemical analysis since it was first separately described in 1946 by Bloch *et al.* (2) and Purcell *et al.* (3). It is only in the last two decades that the biological applications of MRS have become apparent. In 1973 Moon and Richards first studied suspensions of red blood cells (4), and studies of cells, tissues, and isolated organs soon followed. The technological innovations that permitted the introduction of larger and more powerful superconducting magnets into clinical practice allowed the study of human organs *in vivo*. Neonatal brain studies were reported in 1983 (5).

The technique of MRS relies on the magnetic properties of certain nuclei, such as phosphorus-31, that align in a strong uniform magnetic field. These nuclei, within the background magnetic field, emit a radiofrequency (RF) signal when stimulated at their particular resonance frequency. This signal has a *frequency* that is determined by the molecular environment of the ^{31}P nucleus, so different phosphorus-containing compounds can be separated on the basis of their very slightly different resonance frequencies (chemical shifts). The signal also has an *amplitude* which is determined by the number of phosphorus nuclei resonating at any one frequency, and can be used to determine the molar concentration of the different phosphorus-containing compounds (6).

The spectrum shown in Fig. 1A was obtained from a healthy 3-day-old infant. The spectrum was recorded over a period of about 5 min while the baby slept within the 1.9-tesla superconducting magnet of a Bruker Biospec spectrometer. Radiofrequency pulses of 275 μs duration at 3-sec intervals were transmitted from an RF coil beneath the side of the baby's head, and the resulting sequence of MR signals was detected by a 6.5 cm receiver coil. This coil collected MR signals from a large volume of one cerebral hemisphere, and these raw signals were summed and Fourier transformed to provide a frequency spectrum. No sedation or medication is needed for MRS studies, which do not involve ionizing radiation. However, there are major logistic difficulties in studying sick, and especially ventilated, infants in a powerful magnetic field. If iatrogenic disasters are to be avoided, very strict attention to patient safety is needed.

Figure 1A shows the seven peaks seen in the spectrum from a normal brain. Peaks 1, 2, and 3 are predominantly beta, alpha, and gamma adenosine triphosphate (ATP), respectively, peak 5 is attributed to phospholipid bilayers and phosphodiesters (PDE), and peak 7 is phosphomonoester (PME), mainly phosphoethanolamine. The other two peaks are of more importance in assessing cerebral energy status. Peak 4 is phosphocreatine (PCr), and peak 6 (shaded) is inorganic orthophosphate (Pi). When cerebral oxygenation is significantly compromised ATP levels are maintained at the expense of the hydrolysis of PCr. This leads to a fall in PCr levels and a reciprocal rise in Pi, as shown in Fig. 1B from a severely asphyxiated infant, studied at 9 days of age. ATP levels are maintained in all but the most severely asphyxiated infants and ATP depletion is associated with a very poor prognosis.

The time sequence of changes following birth asphyxia is interesting, because spectra recorded in the first 12–24 h show that when a baby is stable following initial resuscitation, cerebral energy status (as reflected by the PCr/Pi ratio) is normal. There is a secondary deterioration of energy metabolism, reaching its nadir at 3–4 days, which is supportive evidence for two-phase cellular injury following brain ischemia (7).

MRS data, and particularly PCr/Pi ratios, have been shown to have major prognostic significance in newborn infants following episodes of cerebral ischemia. In a study of 61 such infants, Azzopardi *et al.* (8) showed that a PCr/Pi ratio below the 95% confidence limits for normal infants predicted death or severe neurological deficit with a sensitivity of only 68% but a specificity of 95% and a positive predictive value of 96%. In practice, therefore, an abnormal PCr/Pi ratio is highly predictive, but a normal PCr/Pi is not necessarily reassuring.

The relatively poor sensitivity of conventional MRS (which is especially evident

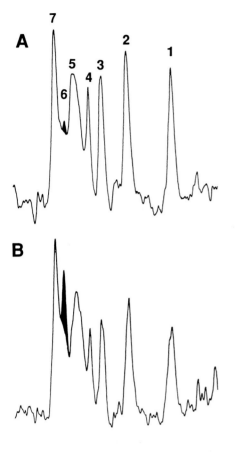

FIG. 1. A: Global MR spectrum from a normal 3-day-old infant. Horizontal frequency axis separates phosphorus metabolites on the basis of their different resonance frequencies. Peak areas correspond to metabolite concentrations. Inorganic phosphate peak is shaded. See text for peak assignments. **B**: Global MR spectrum from a 9-day-old infant following severe birth asphyxia. Inorganic phosphate peak is shaded. (Unpublished spectra from J. Moorcraft, N. M. Bolas, N. K. Ives, P. Sutton, B. Rajagopalan, M. Blackledge, P. L. Hope, and G. K. Radda.)

in those infants who subsequently develop pure motor deficits) may partly be related to the large volume of tissue interrogated by the surface coil. Signals from superficial tissues tend to dominate the "global spectrum" recorded in the classical MRS experiment, and areas of significant energy impairment may be missed, especially if they are deeper in the brain, for instance in periventricular white matter.

Recent work we have carried out in Oxford, in collaboration with Professor Radda's department, has tried to overcome this deficiency by using an MRS technique called phase-modulated rotating frame imaging (PMRFI). PMRFI uses a linear gradient in the RF field to obtain depth-resolved MR spectra, which permits noninvasive biochemical analysis of sequential discs of cerebral tissue about 0.6–1 cm in depth (9). Figure 2, obtained with the help of Bheeshma Rajagopalan, Martin Blackledge, and Nick Bolas, shows three spectra from the same asphyxiated infant whose global spectrum is shown in Fig. 1B. The spectra are from increasing depth into brain tissue.

PMRFI has confirmed that energy impairment following asphyxia is greater at 1–1.5 cm below the brain surface than in more superficial regions, adding support to

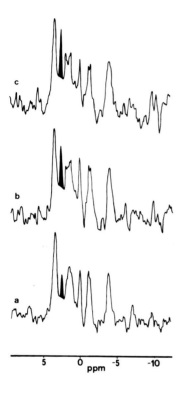

FIG. 2. Depth-resolved MR spectra from the asphyxiated infant whose global spectrum is shown in Fig. 1B, obtained using PMRFI. Spectrum *a* is derived from superficial brain, spectra *b* and *c* from brain 1–2 cm and 2–3 cm below the brain surface, respectively. For technical reasons Peak 1 (β-ATP) is not visible on PMRFI spectra. Inorganic phosphate peak is shaded. Unpublished spectra from J. Moorcraft, N. M. Bolas, N. K. Ives, P. Sutton, B. Rajagopalan, M. Blackledge, P. L. Hope, and G. K. Radda.

the suggestion that subcortical white matter, especially the base of the sulci, is a zone of vascular watershed in the full-term brain (10). Follow-up studies of infants studied by both conventional MRS and PMRFI are at an early stage. Preliminary results show that depth-resolved data are no more predictive than global data in a population of asphyxiated full-term infants. Because damage to periventricular white matter is more common in preterm infants, it may be that PMRFI will have a particular role in assessment of ischemic damage of the preterm brain.

Future potential developments of MRS as a tool for the investigation of the newborn include the study of organs other than the brain, the sophistication of spatial localization techniques, and the study of nuclei other than phosphorus. PMRFI permits study of the liver and heart, because it facilitates the exclusion of MRS signals from overlying muscle. If problems of increased ambient noise and of signal-to-noise ratio can be overcome then combined imaging/spectroscopy systems will allow spectra to be obtained from specific anatomical regions of brain defined by using a cursor on the proton image. Of the alternative nuclei, the technique likely to be of most clinical value is high-resolution proton spectroscopy with water suppression, which has already been used to measure cerebral intracellular lactate concentrations.

MRS has proved a useful research tool for the noninvasive investigation of intracellular biochemistry, and has clinical potential as a prognostic tool. However, there are considerable logistic problems with the technique that preclude its widespread application as a method for general use in clinical neonatology. It is very labor intensive, time-consuming, and requires infants to be transported to the superconducting magnet. The study of sick and ventilator-dependent infants is difficult, and involves considerable patient disturbance and customized apparatus without ferrous metallic components. These limitations were the main stimulus toward the development of alternative technologies for the assessment of cerebral hypoxia-ischemia in neonates requiring intensive care. One such potentially important bedside technique is near-infrared spectroscopy (NIRS).

NEAR-INFRARED SPECTROSCOPY

Living tissues are easily penetrated by light in the near-infrared part of the spectrum (wavelength 700–1,000 nm) and this property has been exploited in near-infrared spectroscopy (NIRS). Three major biological pigments, or chromophores, have characteristic absorption spectra for near-infrared light. These are oxyhemoglobin, deoxyhemoglobin, and oxidized cytochrome aa_3, the terminal enzyme in the mitochondrial electron transport chain. If the absorption characteristics of these three compounds are known, then the attenuation of near-infrared light at three or more wavelengths during its passage through living tissues can be used to calculate the amount of each chromophore in the light path.

Although NIR light passes through brain tissue much more readily than visible light, the loss in intensity is still approximately one order of magnitude per centimeter of tissue. The development of clinically useful systems has therefore relied on the use of high-powered pulsed-laser diodes to produce NIR light at very specific wavelengths, and sensitive photomultipliers operating in photon-counting mode for the detection of the transmitted light. Current technology allows measurements to be made by transmission spectroscopy across heads of 8-cm width using an average power output of 16 mW, which is an order of magnitude below recommended exposure limits. Larger heads can be studied using reflectance spectroscopy, but quantitation of results is less straightforward.

NIRS was pioneered by Franz Jobsis in North Carolina, who first reported studies of animal brains, and a preliminary human experiment in 1977 (11). His NIR spectrometer, marketed as the NIROS-SCOPE, was used in the first study of neonatal brains to be published from Duke University in 1985, by Brazy, Jobsis, and others (12). They described the derivation from animal experiments of the algorithms used to generate the on-line signals corresponding to amounts of oxy- and deoxyhemoglobin and cytochrome aa_3 in the light path, as well as a derived value of tissue blood volume. The paper reports the use of this system to display these cerebral hemodynamic variables in real time at the bedside, and to observe the perturbations caused by changes in the infant's ventilatory status. Quantitation was not attempted in this study.

Further longitudinal monitoring studies have been reported by the group working under Professor Osmund Reynolds and David Delpy at University College Hospital

Block Diagram of the System

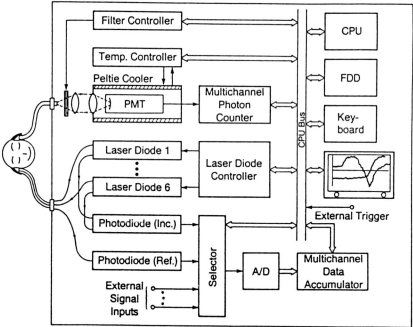

FIG. 3. Block diagram of near-infrared spectroscopy system. (Reproduced from the manufacturer's specifications, with permission of Hamamatsu Photonics Ltd.)

(UCH) in London (13). The UCH group has used a spectrometer developed in cooperation with a Japanese firm, Hamamatsu Photonics, diagrammatically represented in Fig. 3 (14). Figure 4A shows the effects on cerebral hemodynamics of an episode of desaturation in a preterm infant, as demonstrated by NIRS. Figure 4B shows the rise in oxyhemoglobin and oxidized cytochrome aa_3 that occurred in the brain of the same infant in response to a rise in pCO_2.

The UCH group has also developed quantitative analysis, by using NIRS measurements to derive absolute values for cerebral blood flow, cerebral blood volume, and CO_2 reactivity (15). These developments mean that NIRS can be used to derive comparable data from different infants, rather than just measure relative changes longitudinally in single patients.

Absolute quantitation depends on knowledge of the path length of photons between source and sensor, which is considerably complicated by the effect of scattering. A value of 4.3 times the head width has been calculated as the path length by mathematical modelling, and this has been confirmed by "time of flight" measurements using ultrashort pulses of light and a "streak camera" (16).

Cerebral blood volume (CBV) in ml/100 g brain tissue can be calculated from

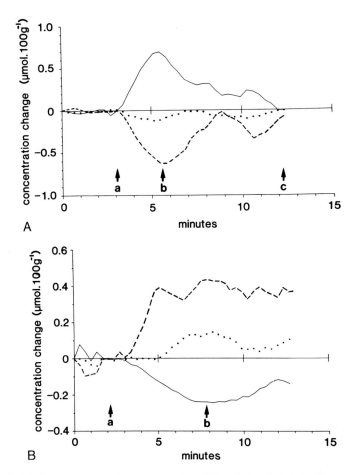

FIG. 4. **A**: NIRS measurements from a 27-week gestation, 1-day-old infant with no cerebral abnormality. $----$, Oxyhemoglobin; ————, deoxyhemoglobin; $\cdots\cdots$, oxidized cytochrome aa₃. Transient decrease in arterial oxygen saturation [96% at *a* and *c*, 84% at *b*. **B**: Further NIRS measurements from the same infant as in **A**, during an increase in pCO₂ from 4.6 kPa to 5.7 kPa between *a* and *b*. (Data from E. O. R. Reynolds, J. S. Wyatt, D. Azzopardi, D. T. Delpy, E. B. Cady, M. Cope, S. Wray, *Br Med Bull* 1988;44:1052–75, with permission.)]

measuring the effect on oxy- and deoxyhemoglobin of a small gradual change in arterial oxygen saturation. CBV has been noted to increase following birth asphyxia, presumably due to accumulation of cerebral vasodilators. CO_2 reactivity of the cerebral circulation, as measured by the change in cerebral blood volume resulting from a known change in arterial pCO₂, also falls following birth asphyxia, perhaps because of maximal cerebral arteriolar vasodilatation. Recently Edwards and the UCH group (17) have reported the use of NIRS to measure cerebral blood flow by an adaptation of the Fick principle. Oxygen is used as the tracer, and the input function is detected by an adapted pulse oximeter on the ear. The arrival of the pulse of oxygen in the brain is detected by NIRS, and the values for cerebral blood flow obtained are consistent with values obtained using radioactive tracer methods.

These techniques have been used to show a prolonged and significant fall in cerebral blood flow following the administration of indomethacin to preterm infants for the medical closure of the patent ductus arteriosus. As well as monitoring the effect of other drugs, interventions, and diseases that may alter cerebral hemodynamics, NIRS may develop a diagnostic and prognostic role in the asphyxiated full-term infant. Cerebrovascular events in the first 24 h of life may be of major importance in the pathogenesis of the secondary energy failure demonstrated by MRS. NIRS may prove useful for the detection of a particularly high-risk group of infants and monitoring of new treatments in this period.

There are obvious attractions to bedside monitoring of cerebral oxygenation, and NIR spectrometers are now in commercial production. The NIR light is transmitted to and from the infant's head by fiberoptic cables attached to small "optodes" which are attached to each temporal region. There is relatively minor disturbance of the infant, but exclusion of ambient light is absolutely essential and the head has to be wrapped with a light-occluding cloth. Measurements are difficult in a struggling baby, and a considerable amount of "postprocessing" of the data on a separate microcomputer is currently necessary to obtain the derived values discussed above. NIRS is still basically a research tool. It will be interesting to see whether its clinical value is proven over the next few years, in which case further generations of spectrometers with more specific software should make NIRS more clinically accessible.

The advent of MRS and NIRS has added considerably to the range of available techniques for the objective assessment of the hypoxic-ischemic neonatal brain. NIRS measures cerebral oxygenation and by measuring oxidized cytochrome aa_3 also reflects intracellular oxygen availability. MRS measures intracellular concentrations of the high-energy phosphorus compounds ATP and PCr, which become depleted following severe hypoxia. The combination of the two should permit valuable noninvasive insights into the mechanisms of neuronal damage following cerebral hypoxia-ischemia. They may point the way to possible therapeutic maneuvers, and should also be useful tools for the objective assessment of the effect of such interventions.

ACKNOWLEDGMENT

Dr. Moorcraft is funded by Action Research.

REFERENCES

1. Hope PL, Gould SJ, Howard S, Hamilton PA, Costello AM deL, Reynolds EOR. Precision of ultrasound diagnosis of pathologically verified lesions in the brains of very preterm infants. *Dev Med Child Neurol* 1988;30:457–71.
2. Bloch F, Hansen WW, Packard ME. Nuclear induction. *Phys Rev* 1946;69:127.

3. Purcell EM, Torrey HC, Pound RV. Resonance absorption by nuclear magnetic moments in a solid. *Phys Rev* 1946;69:37–8.
4. Moon RB, Richards JH. Determination of intracellular pH by 31P magnetic resonance. *J Biol Chem* 1973;248:7276–8.
5. Cady EB, Costello AM deL, Dawson MJ, *et al.* Non-invasive investigation of cerebral metabolism in newborn infants by phosphorus nuclear magnetic resonance spectroscopy. *Lancet* 1983;i:1059–62.
6. Gadian DG. *Nuclear magnetic resonance and its application to living systems.* Oxford: Clarendon Press, 1980.
7. Hope PL, Costello AM deL, Cady EB, *et al.* Cerebral energy metabolism studied with phosphorus NMR spectroscopy in normal and birth-asphyxiated infants. *Lancet* 1984;ii:366–70.
8. Azzopardi D, Wyatt JS, Cady EB, *et al.* Prognosis of newborn infants with hypoxic-ischemic brain injury assessed by phosphorus magnetic resonance spectroscopy. *Pediatr Res* 1989;25:445–51.
9. Blackledge MJ, Rajagopalan B, Oberhaensli RD, *et al.* Quantitative studies of human cardiac metabolism by 31P rotating frame NMR. *Proc Natl Acad Sci USA* 1987;84:4283–7.
10. Takashima S, Armstrong DL, Becker LE. Subcortical leukomalacia. Relationship to development of the cerebral sulcus and its vascular supply. *Arch Neurol* 1978;35:470–2.
11. Jobsis FF. Noninvasive infrared monitoring of cerebral and myocardial oxygen sufficiency and circulatory parameters. *Science* 1977;198:1264–7.
12. Brazy JE, Lewis DV, Mitnick MH, Jobsis van der Vliet F. Noninvasive monitoring of cerebral oxygenation in preterm infants: preliminary observations. *Paediatrics* 1985;75:217–25.
13. Wyatt JS, Cope M, Delpy DT, Wray S, Reynolds EOR. Quantitation of cerebral oxygenation and haemodynamics in sick newborn infants by near infrared spectroscopy. *Lancet* 1986;ii:1063–6.
14. Delpy DT, Cope MC, Cady EB, *et al.* Cerebral monitoring in newborn infants by magnetic resonance and near infrared spectroscopy. *Scand J Clin Lab Invest* 1987;47(Suppl 188):9–17.
15. Wyatt JS, Edwards AD, Azzopardi D, Reynolds EOR. Magnetic resonance and near infrared spectroscopy for investigation of perinatal hypoxic-ischaemic brain injury. *Arch Dis Child* 1989;64:953–63.
16. Delpy DT, Cope M, van der Zee P, Arridge S, Wray S, Wyatt JS. Estimation of optical pathlength through tissue from direct time of flight measurement. *Phys Med Biol* 1988;33:1433–42.
17. Edwards AD, Wyatt JS, Richardson C, Delpy DT, Cope M, Reynolds EOR. Cotside measurement of cerebral blood flow in ill newborn infants by near infrared spectroscopy. *Lancet* 1988;ii:770–1.

DISCUSSION

Dr. Roloff: Those of us who do ECMO may wish to have this machine in our unit in order to have the method available for research on tolerance of hypoxic insults.

Dr. Hope: There are many things to look at, and we are starting with more traditional therapies. There are numerous questions still to be answered about the use of inotropes in the preterm infant, and about the degree of volume loading necessary to achieve cerebral perfusion. These are clinical problems that we face every day and I think we still largely work on prejudice. One of the interventions we perform about which there has been much concern is the use of indomethacin, which has been shown both on Doppler and more recently on NIRS to be associated with a considerable and sustained fall in cerebral blood flow, whether it is given by bolus or by continuous slow infusion. So there are many interventions to test including, perhaps, ECMO in the long term.

Dr. Roloff: Do you find that treatment methods we ordinarily consider as indicated to improve oxygenation may result in decreased tissue oxygenation while PO_2 or other accepted measures of oxygenation improve?

Dr. Hope: Certainly. Skin oxygenation, for example, may be a poor indicator of brain oxygenation. If we could demonstrate satisfactory cerebral oxygenation at lowish pO_2 values, maybe we could avoid unnecessary barotrauma in some preterm infants.

Dr. Holzgreve: Can the technique be used to identify placental infarction, particularly in the anterior wall, which is close to the surface of the maternal abdomen?

Dr. Hope: It is a major problem to look at tissues more than a few millimeters or maybe a centimeter deep. Light intensity falls exponentially with depth so the majority of the NIR signal will come from the maternal abdominal wall. People have looked at the placenta with magnetic resonance spectroscopy and this is feasible with an anterior placenta.

Dr. Rosén: Is there a possibility of using deep frozen specimens for magnetic resonance analysis?

Dr. Hope: It is increasingly realized that even the most sophisticated freeze-clamping results in degradation, especially of phosphocreatine. Especially in larger organs, where freezing is not instantaneous, freeze clamping is probably rather less accurate than *in vivo* MRS.

Dr. Merchant: Are there any data, either with NMR or infrared, to assess the effectiveness of therapy? Have any infrared studies been done after therapy for asphyxia in experimental animals?

Dr. Hope: Some studies have been done but they are very difficult. At University College Hospital we looked at the effect of mannitol infusions in asphyxiated infants in whom ultrasound examination suggested cerebral edema. There was no immediate effect on cerebral energy metabolism in the 30 min following a standard bolus of mannitol. Experimental studies involving the survival and recovery of severely asphyxiated animals are very difficult and in Oxford we are currently limited in our ability to study neonates sequentially because our magnet is in a different building.

Dr. Merchant: If such data were available one would have extremely strong evidence to show which forms of therapy are most effective in cerebral edema and asphyxia.

Dr. Hope: There are exciting prospects in terms of therapy, particularly the use of calcium entry blockers and antagonists of excitatory neurotransmitters.

Dr. Caccamo: How long does an NMR examination last? Is an anesthetic necessary?

Dr. Hope: No. Most neonates lie still after a feed. The global spectrum takes 5–10 min and the full PMFR "image" takes about 20–30 min.

Dr. Dawes: That length of time bothers me because you can expect a change of energy distribution in the brain during sleep cycles, particularly in the brain stem nuclei. Is there a possibility of shorter measurement periods?

Dr. Hope: The signal-to-noise ratio is dependent on field strength; a higher field strength improves sensitivity. However, there is the important issue of biological safety. The current recommended upper limit of field strength is 2.5 tesla, i.e., just above the value of 1.9 tesla that we are using. By the time one reaches 4 tesla and above, biological effects such as induced potentials in the field are more likely. If we can't increase the magnet strength, then at least a few minutes of measurement are required to obtain acceptable signal-to-noise ratio to get the global spectrum, and longer to use any of the current techniques of spatial localization. I should like to ask whether you think the sort of energy failure we see is likely to occur during sleep cycles. Our technique tells us about severe brain injury but I should be surprised if energy metabolism was deranged and phosphocreatine depleted during sleep cycles.

Dr. Dawes: That is a perfectly good question and the answer is no. You are probably dealing with degradation of energy reserves far greater than normal.

Perinatology, edited by Erich Saling,
Nestlé Nutrition Workshop Series, Vol. 26,
Nestec, Ltd., Vevey/Raven Press, Ltd.,
New York © 1992.

Surfactant Replacement Therapy: Benefits and Risks

Tetsuro Fujiwara, Shoichi Chida, and Mineo Konishi

Department of Pediatrics, Iwate Medical University School of Medicine, Uchimaru 19-I, Morioka 020, Iwate, Japan

Surfactant deficiency at birth makes it difficult for the newborn to inflate its lungs. As the infant makes increasingly vigorous attempts to ventilate noncompliant lungs, delayed adsorption of lung fluid, pulmonary edema, extravasation of plasma proteins into air spaces, and lung injury occur, which cause progressive respiratory distress. Intratracheal administration of surfactant into the infant's lungs is a reasonable approach to replenish the missing surfactant.

Exogenous surfactant preparations of various types have now been evaluated in treatment of established respiratory distress syndrome (RDS) and to prevent its development. Since our initial report in 1980 (1), there have been a number of controlled studies reporting the efficacy of surfactant preparations of various types, and other trials are ongoing around the world. The prospect of surfactant therapy for premature infants is now reaching an exciting stage.

This chapter provides an overview of the available surfactant preparations for clinical use, the currently reported results, the clinical implications of such therapy on the course of RDS, and some risk versus benefit considerations.

SURFACTANT PREPARATIONS FOR CLINICAL USE

It is useful to group the available surfactant preparations into three categories. The first consists of an organic solvent extract of animal lung lavage or of minced lung saline extract with or without additives. The second is natural surfactant isolated from human amniotic fluid. Thirdly, there are artificial or synthetic surfactants (Table 1).

CLINICAL EFFICACY OF SURFACTANT PREPARATIONS

It is useful to group the reported trials of surfactant therapy into two categories: rescue trials and prophylactic trials. Rescue trials have used surfactants to treat

TABLE 1. *Published randomized clinical trials of surfactants in infants with RDS*

Strategy	Study	Surfactant	Dose[a]	Response	Duration
Prevention	Halliday *et al.* (2)	DPPC/HDL	30 mg	Negligible	—
	Enhorning *et al.* (3)	Infasurf	75–100 mg	Striking	Sustained
	Kwong *et al.* (4)	CLSE	90 mg	Striking	Sustained
	Shapiro *et al.* (5)	CLSE	90 mg	Striking	Unsustained
	Merritt *et al.* (6)	Human AFS	multiple	Striking	Sustained
	Ten Centre (7)	ALEC	multiple	Not studied	—
	Kendig *et al.* (8)	CLSE	90 mg	Striking	Unsustained
Rescue	Wilkinson *et al.* (9)	ALEC	25 mg	Negligible	—
	Hallman *et al.* (10)	Human AFS	multiple	Striking	Sustained
	Gitlin *et al.* (11)	Surfactant TA	120 mg	Striking	Sustained
	Raju *et al.* (12)	Surfactant TA	120 mg	Striking	Sustained
	Fujiwara *et al.* (13)	Surfactant TA	120 mg	Striking	Sustained
	McCord *et al.* (14)	Curosurf	200 mg	Striking	Sustained
	CEMSG (15)	Curosurf	200 mg	Striking	Sustained
	Horbar *et al.* (16)	Survanta	120 mg	Striking	Sustained

[a] Total lipid/kg body weight.
AFS, amniotic fluid surfactant; ALEC, artificial lung expanding compound (DPPC:phosphatidyl-glycerol, 7:3); CEMSG, Collaborative European Multicentre Study Group; CLSE, calf lung lavage surfactant lipid extract; Curosurf, phospholipid fraction of porcine lung extract; DPPC, dipalmitoylphosphatidylcho-line; HDL, high-density lipoprotein; Infasurf, cow lung lavage surfactant lipid (additive, $CaCl_2$); Surfactant TA, a reconstituted bovine lung surfactant lipid (additives, DPPC, tripalmitin, and palmitic acid); Survanta, a modification of Surfactant TA.
Sustained effect lasts for at least 48 h after administration of surfactant.
From Fujiwara T, *et al.* (13).

infants with established RDS, whereas prophylactic trials have used surfactants before the infant's first breath or within minutes of delivery to modify the course of RDS in infants at high risk of RDS. Many of the therapeutic benefits of various naturally derived surfactant preparations in RDS have been described in a series of recent, randomized trials, all of which showed statistically significant improvements in respiratory function after surfactant therapy. However, the immediate physiologic responses achieved with naturally derived surfactants have not been reproduced with the currently reported synthetic surfactants (2,7,17).

Mechanical ventilator usage and initial ventilator settings vary from one study to another, but our protocol (13,18) includes initial ventilator settings of 20–30 breaths/min, positive inspiratory pressures of 20–30 cm H_2O, positive end-expiratory pressures of 4 cm H_2O, and inspiratory duration of 1.0, which are optimal for most RDS patients weighing less than 1,750 g. After treatment FiO_2 is reduced, followed by reductions in peak pressures and ventilator rates. The FiO_2 can usually be reduced to less than 0.3 to 0.4 by 1 hour when treated within 30 min of birth and by 3 hours when treated at 6 hours of age, and an accelerated course of weaning from a mechanical ventilation can be accomplished. Figure 1 illustrates improvements in oxygenation and ventilatory requirement of RDS patients weighing 750–1249 g following treatment with surfactant TA.

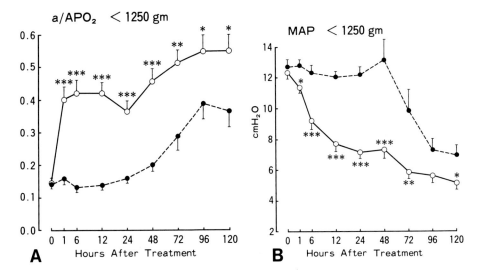

FIG. 1. Sequential values of arterial/alveolar oxygen tension ratio (a/APO₂) (**A**) and mean airway pressure (MAP) (**B**) of RDS patients weighing 750-1,249 g following surfactant treatment. O—O, Surfactant TA ($n = 23$); ●--●, air placebo ($n = 19$). Age at treatment: surfactant, 5.5 h; placebo, 4.8 h. Mean ± SE. *$p < 0.05$, **$p < 0.01$, ***$p < 0.001$ (Wilcoxon rank sum test, two-tailed). Reprinted with permission from ref. 13.

In most trials surfactant preparations have been evaluated in comparison with conventionally ventilated infants from 23 to 30 weeks' gestation. However, most study designs have not required that premature infants treated with surfactant have evidence of surfactant deficiency. Surfactant deficiency was documented in only five (6,9,10,13,18) of the 16 clinical trials reported to date either through a biochemical measure of lung maturity (i.e., lecithin-to-sphingomyelin ratio) in amniotic fluid (6,9,10), or by biophysical analysis of surfactant (stable microbubble rating (19) in gastric aspirates obtained at birth (13,18). Patient selection is a key factor because of the higher frequency of mature lung function among infants (40–60%) of <30 weeks' gestation. A prophylactic strategy is a reasonable approach only when the infant has surfactant deficiency. Unfortunately, it is not always known which infants have surfactant deficiency. Perhaps definite lung immaturity justifies prophylactic surfactant strategy.

Studies with human amniotic fluid surfactant have shown a nonsustained response in 41% of infants with established RDS and in 71% of infants treated prophylactically. In both of these studies (6,10) infants needed multiple doses of surfactant to sustain the therapeutic response. In contrast to the prophylactic trial by Enhorning *et al.* (3), a recent similar trial using a single dose of CLSE (calf lung lavage extract) showed that the effects diminished between 24 and 48 h after surfactant administration (8).

By and large, study groups in different clinical trials reported to date have not been comparable, and the question as to optimal timing of surfactant therapy remains unanswered. The reason for the variation in response and for the nonresponse in some infants has not been clarified. Besides demographic variation, many factors may account for such variation in response, including a multitude of routine practices, approach to the management of patent ductus arteriosus, severity of RDS, differences in conventional ventilatory techniques, variations in the dose of surfactant, or variability in biophysical and physiologic activity among the different surfactant preparations.

The important issue regarding the correlation between the *in vitro* surface properties and *in vivo* surface properties has been extensively studied by Notter (20). A major concern about naturally derived surfactants (amniotic fluid surfactant, CLSE, or porcine surfactant) has been related to quality control. Natural surfactant obtained by lung lavage contains various forms of phospholipid micelles with different surface active properties (21) and different metabolic characteristics (22). Recent studies from our laboratory (23) demonstrated striking differences between Surfactant TA and other naturally derived or synthetic surfactants with respect to the minimal quantity required to display the acceptable *in vitro* surface active properties, the capability of forming stable microbubbles (diameter <15 mμ), and microstructures. These studies suggest that treatment with preparations rich in the less surface-active components relative to the active components would require a larger dose to have an equivalent clinical response to that seen with surfactant rich in the more surface-active components.

Another important factor recently recognized is the variability in sensitivity of surfactants to alveolar protein inhibitors. Surfactant TA is quite resistant to alveolar protein inhibitors as compared with other surfactants (24). It is unclear whether infants having a more favorable response to surfactant release less inhibitor, have lower effluent protein concentrations, or both. *In vitro* studies suggest that a higher dose of surfactant can overcome the inhibitory effects of plasma components on surfactant (25).

Most of the trials reported to date have shown that although there is a statistically significant benefit of surfactant treatment in decreasing the severity of RDS when compared with controls, the majority of the infants still suffer from the disease. In prospective randomized (13,18) and nonrandomized (26) trials, we have shown that the majority of surfactant recipients require minimal ventilatory support equivalent to that of most ventilated preterm infants without parenchymal lung disease. Optimal response seen in this group of infants may typify the response in "pure" RDS, in which surfactant deficiency is the primary factor. On the other hand, suboptimal response (ventilatory index >0.03 or FiO$_2$ >0.3 and MAP >6 cm H$_2$O) seen in some of the surfactant recipients are related to several factors: (a) some degree of early lung injury due to surfactant deficiency occurring before surfactant therapy (27); (b) increased alveolar capillary permeability and secondary surfactant inactivation by proteins leaking into the alveolar space (28); (c) some degree of structural immaturity; or (d) pathophysiologic conditions of RDS other than surfactant deficiency (26,29). Recent clinical and experimental evidence suggests that some of these factors affecting the response to surfactant can be eliminated by treating at birth (3), sooner after birth (30), increasing dosage (18), and/or using a multiple-dose strategy (31).

Clinical trials comparing the prophylactic or very early versus rescue strategies are in progress.

EFFECT OF SURFACTANT THERAPY ON COMPLICATIONS OF RDS

The surfactant therapy eliminates the surfactant deficiency component of the complex pathophysiology of RDS (26). Since surfactant therapy reduces the severity of RDS and restores sufficient lung function to permit a reduction in ventilatory support (lower FiO_2 and lower mean airway pressures), one might predict that surfactant therapy will reduce the major morbidity factors of RDS such as air leaks, bronchopulmonary dysplasia (BPD), and intracranial hemorrhage (ICH). The controlled clinical trials of both prophylactic and rescue types reported the substantial reduction in the frequency of the major complications of RDS. These trials are not equivalent, yet they are sufficiently similar for us to have summed the complications across studies as shown below.

Prophylactic Trials

To date, 104 infants have been treated prophylactically in three controlled trials with naturally derived surfactants, which have shown a significant impact on the complications of RDS and prematurity (Fig. 2). Estimates derived from 95% confidence intervals (CI) are that pneumothorax decreases by between 7% and 28% ($p = 0.003$), and pulmonary interstitial emphysema (PIE) decreases by between 18% and 40% ($p<0.001$). There was no statistically significant reduction in the frequency of ICH and BPD. The 95% CI for the overall increase in survival in the group treated prophylactically was between 2% and 31% ($p = 0.009$). Of the prophylactic trials, those of Enhorning *et al.* (3) and Merritt *et al.* (6) showed a substantial reduction in mortality. In recent prophylactic trials (17) using a saline suspension of the DPPC/PG mixture, the beneficial effect on gas exchange was found to begin 18 h after multiple-dose treatments, associated with a substantial reduction in ICH and morbidity.

Rescue Trials

In the rescue trials, 262 infants have been treated (Fig. 3). The incidence of pneumothorax or PIE was also significantly reduced.

In contrast to prophylactic trials, the frequency of ICH decreased significantly from 47% to 37%, with a 95% CI of between 1% and 18% ($p = 0.043$). In the two Japanese rescue trials (13,18) reporting a significant decrease of ICH, the study designs have required the absence of ultrasonographic evidence of $\geq$ grade 2 ICH at randomization, and the timing of occurrence of hemorrhage during the study period was determined in a prospective fashion using scheduled cranial ultrasonographic

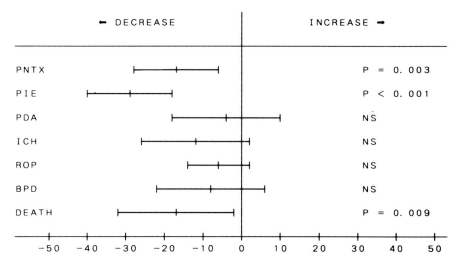

FIG. 2. Effects of "prevention" surfactant therapy on complications of RDS. The complications were summed (see text) across the studies reported by Enhorning *et al.* (3), Merritt *et al.* (6), and Kendig *et al.* (8) who used naturally derived surfactant preparations. PNTX, pneumothorax; PIE, pulmonary interstitial emphysema; PDA, patent ductus arteriosus; ICH, intracranial hemorrhage; ROP, retinopathy of prematurity; BPD, bronchopulmonary dysplasia. Probability of less than 0.05 by Fisher exact test (two-tailed) was considered significant; 95% confidence intervals for difference in incidence.

scans. Since any ICH may occur very early, i.e., within a few hours of birth (32,33) some infants with such early hemorrhage might have been enrolled in trials in which no beneficial effect of surfactant on hemorrhage was found. Unless ultrasonographic scans were performed on all infants at delivery, none of the prophylactic studies can provide documentation of prestudy ICH status at birth.

The reduction in the frequency of BPD was marginally significant ($p = 0.056$), and between 3% and 22% ($p = 0.008$) more infants survived. Of these trials, that of Raju *et al.* (12), using a single 120 mg/kg dose of Surfactant TA, observed a reduction in mortality from 54% for the control group to 18% for the treated infants. The collaborative European multicenter study group (15), using a single 200 mg/kg dose of Curosurf, also observed a reduction in mortality from 51% to 31% when treated infants were compared with controls. In both of these studies, the death rate in control infants was much higher than the 17–26% observed in other studies. Different patient selection criteria may have contributed to the differences in outcome among the studies.

Potential Risk

Remarkably little adverse effect (or toxicity) has become apparent in the animal and clinical studies of surfactant (34).

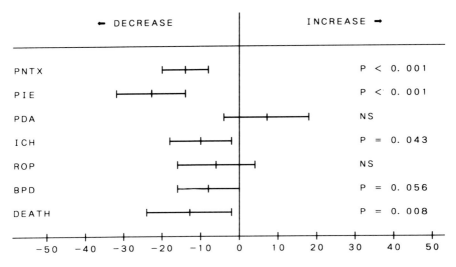

FIG. 3. Effects of "rescue" surfactant therapy on complications of RDS. The complications were summed (see text) across the studies reported by Hallman *et al.* (10), Gitlin *et al.* (11), Raju *et al.* (12), Fujiwara *et al.* (13), collaborative European multicenter study group (15), and Horbar *et al.* (16). Abbreviations and statistical analysis used are the same as in Fig. 2; 95% confidence intervals for difference in incidence.

Although most infants tolerate the intratracheal instillation of liquid surfactant, this unusual route of drug administration is not without risks for a tiny preterm infant; decrease in oxygenation, increase in $PaCO_2$, and some disturbance in systemic blood pressure may occur during the period of administration of surfactant (35). Care must be taken to minimize perturbations in systemic blood pressure and/or cerebral blood flow during surfactant administration. Ventilation with near 100% oxygen and use of longer inspiratory times and slightly higher peak inspiratory pressures during the period of administration of surfactant, along with continuous monitoring of tc-PO_2, $PaCO_2$, and systemic blood pressure, appear helpful (26). Our protocol includes continuous monitoring of systemic blood pressure during the period of administration of surfactant (Fig. 4) and during the subsequent course, in the light of recent work showing that infants at highest risk for ICH can be identified before the onset of hemorrhage by the presence of fluctuations in arterial blood pressure and/or cerebral blood flow velocity (36).

There has been some concern about bovine surfactant because of the presence of a small amount of cow proteolipid apoproteins (1%, SP-B,C), which are the functionally important constituents of exogenous surfactant (37). However, attempts to immunize goats with Surfactant TA by a vigorous hyperimmunization technique that was repeated for 6 months were unsuccessful. We have been unable to detect any antibodies against this protein in more than 600 sera from the 204 patients treated with Surfactant TA (38). Others (39) also were unable to detect antibodies against the proteolipid proteins in 1,202 sera from the 359 patients who were treated with Surfactant TA.

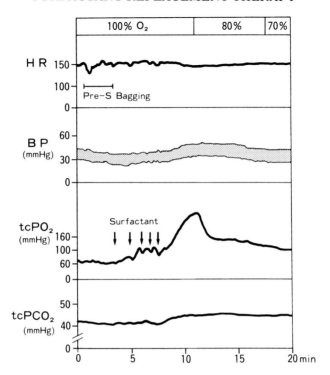

FIG. 4. Continuous tracings of heart rate (beats/min), systemic blood pressures (mm Hg), transcutaneous PO₂ (mm Hg), and transcutaneous PCO₂ (mm Hg) before, during, and after administration of Surfactant TA in an infant with severe RDS (birth weight 860 g, age 6 h), reproduced from the recordings on a Hewlett-Packard monitor (78834A). Pre-S bagging indicates manual bagging when the infant was disconnected from ventilator to have inserted a F-4 feeding tube attached to the syringe containing surfactant through the endotracheal tube. Note that there are no significant changes in heart rate, systolic and diastolic blood pressures, and transcutaneous PCO₂ levels during the period of intratracheal instillation of surfactant and subsequent course.

Liechty *et al.* (40) recently found no differences in the concentrations of plasma atrial natriuretic factor between RDS patients given Salvanta and those given placebo.

Follow-up of Surfactant-Treated Infants

Several studies on follow-up of surfactant-treated infants are in progress around the world. Dunn *et al.* (41) found no differences between the infants given a bovine-based surfactant and control infants with respect to allergic symptoms, respiratory problems, or neurodevelopmental outcome. Vaucher *et al.* (42) demonstrated improved neurodevelopmental performance among infants treated with human surfactant and speculated that decrease in the frequency of BPD should ultimately lead to improved long-term outcome.

SUMMARY

This overview analysis of the current clinical trials of various surfactant preparations suggests that use of these preparations to both prevent and treat RDS should be effective in decreasing major morbidity factors of RDS and mortality. The benefits of such therapy greatly exceed the putative hazards.

The beneficial effects of surfactant therapy have been shown to last for at least 72 h in several studies, but these effects were not consistently seen in other studies. Clinical experience with surfactant treatment, and a little future projection, suggest that the impact on bronchopulmonary dysplasia, intracranial hemorrhage, and mortality should eventually be greater. Using our therapeutic regimen with a single dose Surfactant TA, we have had increased survivors without BPD and/or ICH.

Although we still see some infants with mild BPD, requiring little, or less than 30%, supplemental oxygen, the prevalence of such chronic lung disease in tiny infants treated with surfactant does not differ from that of intubated infants without lung disease, of comparable gestational age and birth weight.

Surfactant therapy unmasks the relative contributions of other mechanisms to the overall spectrum of RDS which include a hemodynamically significant PDA, persistent fetal circulation (clear lung with hypoperfusion), cardiogenic shock, transient myocardial dysfunction with or without tricuspid regurgitation associated with severe perinatal asphyxia, etc. In assessing the effectiveness of surfactant treatment we should consider possible effects of these underlying abnormalities that may complicate the interpretation of the response. Serial-echo and color Doppler echocardiographic examinations are useful in identifying these underlying abnormalities. With early recognition, management, and possible prevention of these circulatory disturbances (PDA, hypotension), it may be possible to increase the significance of surfactant treatment further, and facilitate uncomplicated recovery.

In order to optimize the effects of surfactant therapy, future refinement will also be needed in our understanding of surfactant preparations, instillation techniques including pre- and postsurfactant ventilation, and weaning guidelines, dose, dose schedule, and patient selection.

The isolation and characterization of three surfactant proteins (SP-A, -B and -C) has considerably changed our understanding of the nature and properties of pulmonary surfactant and its metabolism. In the 1990s, we shall have a second or third generation surfactant consisting of synthetic lipids and proteolipid apoproteins (SP-B, -C) that are produced by recombinant DNA technology or direct chemical synthesis.

REFERENCES

1. Fujiwara T, Maeta H, Chida S, Morita T, Watabe Y, Abe N. Artificial surfactant therapy in hyaline membrane disease. *Lancet* 1980;1:55–9.
2. Halliday HL, McClure G, Reid MMc, *et al.* Controlled trial of artificial surfactant to prevent respiratory distress syndrome. *Lancet* 1984;1:476–8.

3. Enhorning G, Shennan A, Possmayer F, Dunn M, Chen CP, Milligan J. Prevention of neonatal respiratory distress syndrome by tracheal instillation of surfactant: a randomized clinical trial. *Pediatrics* 1985;76:145–53.
4. Kwong MS, Eagan EA, Notter RH, Shapiro DL. Double-blind clinical trial of calf lung surfactant extract for the prevention of hyaline membrane disease in extremely premature infants. *Pediatrics* 1985;76:585–92.
5. Shapiro DL, Notter RH, Morin FC III, *et al.* Double-blind randomized trial of a calf lung surfactant extract administered at birth to very premature infants for prevention of respiratory distress syndrome. *Pediatrics* 1985;76:593–9.
6. Merritt A, Hallman M, Bloom BT, *et al.* Prophylactic treatment of very premature infants with human surfactant. *N Engl J Med* 1986;315:785–90.
7. Ten Centre Study Group. Ten centre trial of artificial surfactant (artificial lung expanding compound) in very premature babies. *Br Med J* 1987;294:991–6.
8. Kendig JW, Notter RH, Cox C, *et al.* Surfactant replacement therapy at birth: final analysis of a clinical trial and comparisons with similar trials. *Pediatrics* 1988;82:756–62.
9. Wilkinson A, Jenkins PA, Jeffrey JA. Two controlled trials of dry artificial surfactant: early effects and later outcome in babies with surfactant deficiency. *Lancet* 1985;ii:287–91.
10. Hallman M, Merritt A, Jarvenpaa A-L, *et al.* Exogenous human surfactant for treatment of severe respiratory distress syndrome: a randomized prospective clinical trial. *J Pediatr* 1985;106:963–9.
11. Gitlin JD, Soll RF, Parad RB, *et al.* Randomized controlled trial of exogenous surfactant for the treatment of hyaline membrane disease. *Pediatrics* 1987;79:31–7.
12. Raju TNK, Bhat R, McCulloch KM, *et al.* Double-blind controlled trial of single-dose treatment with bovine surfactant in severe hyaline membrane disease. *Lancet* 1987;i:651–5.
13. Fujiwara T, Konishi M, Nanbu H, *et al.* Surfactant therapy in RDS: results of a multicenter randomized trial. *Jpn J Pediatr* 1987;40:549–68.
14. McCord FB, Curstedt T, Halliday HL, McClure G, Reid MMcC, Robertson B. Surfactant treatment and incidence of intraventricular hemorrhage in severe respiratory distress syndrome. *Arch Dis Child* 1988;63:10–16.
15. Collaborative European Multicenter Study Group. Surfactant replacement therapy for severe neonatal respiratory distress syndrome: an international randomized clinical trial. *Pediatrics* 1988;82:683–91.
16. Horbar JD, Soll RF, Sutherland JM, *et al.* A multicenter randomized, placebo-controlled trial of surfactant therapy for respiratory distress syndrome. *N Engl J Med* 1988;320:959–65.
17. Morley CJ, Greenough A, Miller NG, *et al.* Randomized trial of artificial surfactant (ALEC) given at birth to babies from 23 to 34 weeks gestation. *Early Hum Dev* 1988;17:41–54.
18. Konishi M, Fujiwara T, Naito N, *et al.* Surfactant replacement therapy in neonatal respiratory distress syndrome: a multicenter, randomized clinical trial: comparison of high- vs low-dose of surfactant TA. *Eur J Pediatr* 1987;50:121–9.
19. Pattle RE, Kratzing CC, Parkinson CE, *et al.* Maturity of fetal lungs tested by production of stable microbubbles in amniotic fluid. *Br J Obstet Gynaecol* 1979;86:615–22.
20. Notter RH. Biophysical behavior of lung surfactant: implication for respiratory physiology and pathology. *Semin Perinatol* 1988;12:180–212.
21. Wright JR, Clements JA. State of art: metabolism and turnover of lung surfactant. *Am Rev Respir Dis* 1987;135:426–44.
22. Jobe A, Ikegami M, Seidner SR, Pettenazzo A, Ruffini L. Surfactant phosphatidylcholine metabolism and surfactant function in preterm, ventilated lambs. *Am Rev Respir Dis* 1989;139:352–9.
23. Sasaki M. Comparison of five surfactants: surface properties and electronmicroscopic observations. *Iwate Med J* 1990;42:883–96.
24. Ikegami M, Agata Y, Elkady T, *et al.* Comparison of four surfactants: in vitro surface properties and responses of preterm lambs to treatment at birth. *Pediatrics* 1987;79:38–46.
25. Fuchimukai T, Fujiwara T, Takahasi A, Enhorning G. Artificial pulmonary surfactant inhibited by proteins. *J Appl Physiol* 1987;62:429–39.
26. Fujiwara T, Konishi M, Chida S, Maeta H. Factors affecting the response to a postnatal single dose of a reconstituted bovine surfactant (Surfactant TA). In: Lachman B, ed. *Surfactant replacement therapy in neonatal and adult respiratory distress syndrome.* Berlin: Springer-Verlag, 1989;91–107.
27. Robertson B. Pathology and pathophysiology of neonatal surfactant deficiency. In: Robertson B, Van Golde LMG, Batenburg JJ, eds. *Pulmonary surfactant.* Amsterdam: Elsevier Science Publishers, 1984;383–418.
28. Jobe A, Ikegami M. Surfactant for the treatment of respiratory distress syndrome. *Am Rev Respir Dis* 1987;136:1256–75.

29. Charon A, Taeusch HW Jr, Fitzgibbon C, Smith GB, Treves ST, Phelps DS. Factors associated with surfactant treatment response in infants with severe respiratory distress syndrome. *Pediatrics* 1989;83:348–54.
30. Maeta H, Vidyasagar D, Raju TNK, Bhat R, Matsuda H. Early and late surfactant treatments in baboon model of hyaline membrane disease. *Pediatrics* 1988;81:277–83.
31. Shapiro DL. Comments on dosage and timing of surfactant administration. In: Jobe A, Taeusch HW, eds. *Surfactant treatment of lung disease. Report of the 96th Ross Conference on Pediatric Research.* Columbus, OH: Ross Laboratories, 1988;117–21.
32. Che De Crespiny L, Mackay R, Murton L, Roy RND, Robinson DH. Timing of neonatal cerebro-ventricular haemorrhage with ultrasound. *Arch Dis Child* 1982;57:231–3.
33. Beverley DW, Chance GW, Coates CF. Intraventricular haemorrhage-timing of occurrence and re-lationship to perinatal events. *Br J Obstet Gynaecol* 1984;91:1007–13.
34. Taeusch WH, Alleyne A, Takahashi A, Fan B, Nguyen T, Franco G. Surfactant treatment of res-piratory distress syndrome: selected clinical issues. Creasy RK, Warshaw JB, eds. *Semin Perinatol* 1988;12:245–54.
35. Jorch G, Rabe H, Garbe M, Michel E, Gortner L. Acute and protracted effects of intratracheal surfactant application on internal carotide blood flow velocity, blood pressure and carbon dioxide tension in very low birth weight infants. *Eur J Pediatr* 1989;148:770–3.
36. Perlman JM, McMenahim JB, Volpe JJ. Fluctuating cerebral blood-flow velocity in respiratory dis-tress syndrome. *N Engl J Med* 1983;369:204–9.
37. Possmayer F. A proposed nomenclature for pulmonary surfactant-associated proteins. *Am Rev Respir Dis* 1988;138:990–8.
38. Kawashima T, Chida S, Fujiwara T. Measurements of anti-surfactant proteolipid-5-kDa apoprotein antibodies in sera from HMD-patients treated with surfactant TA using an ELISA. *Perinatal Med (Jpn)* 1987;17:473–6.
39. Hull WH, Whitsett JA. Immunologic analysis of infants receiving surfactant TA. *Pediatr Res* 1988;23:411A.
40. Liechty EA, Johnson MD, Myerberg DZ, Mullett MD. Daily sequential changes in plasma atrial natriuretic factor concentrations in mechanically ventilated low-birth weight infants—effect of sur-factant replacement. *Biol Neonate* 1989;55:244–50.
41. Dunn MS, Shennan AT, Hoskins EM, Lennox K, Enhorning G. Two year follow-up of infants in a randomized trial with surfactant replacement for the prevention of neonatal respiratory distress syn-drome. *Pediatrics* 1988;82:543–7.
42. Vaucher YE, Merritt TA, Hallman M, Jaarvenpaa AL. Neurodevelopmental and respiratory outcome in early childhood after human surfactant treatment. *Am J Dis Child* 1988;142:927–30.

DISCUSSION

Dr. Roloff: Are your trials done with one dose or with multiple doses?

Dr. Fujiwara: At present we use a single dose. We have studied more than 500 patients in our own center and in three multicenter studies involving 50 collaborating centers, and one dose has been used in more than 90% of the patients. A multicenter randomized study comparing single versus multiple doses is under way in Japan.

Dr. Merchant: How do you decide whether to administer surfactant?

Dr. Fujiwara: We have recently completed a randomized clinical trial comparing very early versus late therapy. Inasmuch as the prevalence of RDS in our center is about 35% in babies less than 29 weeks' gestation, we might treat 65% normal babies if all are treated early. We therefore employ a rapid surfactant test, the Pattle stable microbubble test, in gastric aspirates obtained at birth. We have confirmed that this test is as reliable as other established tests such as the L/S ratio or the immunologic quantification of surfactant-associated proteins in predicting RDS. The great advantage is that it only takes 10 min to get a result. We therefore use this test to identify babies in need of early surfactant prophylaxis, and it has been used in all our trials.

Dr. Kienast: If a second dose of surfactant is to be given, what is the preferred interval following the initial dose?

Dr. Fujiwara: We rarely find it necessary to give a second dose but in a few cases we have given one at around 24–36 h of age. This is in contrast to the findings of the Shapiro study. One reason might be that their babies were smaller than ours. Another important variable could be the quality of surfactant used. Quality control of surface activity of the surfactant used is very important, whether single or second dose strategy is used.

Dr. Dawes: You have shown that your kind of surfactant is excellent. The problem I have is understanding why, after such surfactant treatment, some babies still die. Is there another pathological problem within your infant population such as pulmonary hypoplasia? It may be that your surfactant treatment is 95 or 100% effective and that you are underestimating its true performance. Have you a method for measuring independently what is due to lack of surfactant and what is due to pulmonary hypoplasia?

Dr. Fujiwara: Surfactant therapy is not a panacea. Premature babies with RDS have many pathophysiologic conditions besides surfactant deficiency as you rightly point out. The advantage of surfactant therapy is that it not only treats the surfactant deficiency but it also unmasks the relative contribution of several other factors to the complex pathophysiology of RDS. Other problems with oxygenation include transitional fetal circulation and myocardial dysfunction with or without tricuspid regurgitation.

Dr. Marini: One common problem is persistent ductus arteriosus. How do you manage this, and does treatment for PDA reduce the frequency of IVH?

Dr. Fujiwara: In our center we use an oral dose of mefenamic acid, a potent prostaglandin synthetase inhibitor. We found no difference in the frequency of PDA between surfactant-treated and control babies in our multicenter trial. Multiple regression analysis showed no significant interaction between PDA and IVH.

Dr. Marini: In our studies of the "rescue" administration of surfactant we found that there was an immediate and good improvement in gas exchange but pulmonary compliance took much longer to improve. In reptilians there are no alveoli but a lot of surfactant-like material in their bag-like lungs (1). Could surfactant facilitate oxygen transport in ways other than by reducing surface tension?

Dr. Fujiwara: We certainly cannot treat all aspects of the immature lung with surfactant alone. However, treatment with surfactant is also beneficial in restoring pulmonary stability and in reducing ventilator pressures and FiO_2, thereby lessening the incidence of barotrauma, oxygen toxicity, and BPD. IVH is reduced as well because there are fewer risk factors for its occurrence.

Dr. Dawes: I take it that the purpose of giving surfactant is to provide a period during which there is enough surfactant for the newborn lung to start working until the system that normally regulates its supply comes into operation. Have you looked at methods of accelerating the natural process?

Dr. Fujiwara: Dr. Jobe and his associates are testing the efficacy of antenatal treatment with glucocorticoid and thyrotropin releasing hormone in animal models and have found that pretreatment with these hormones enhances the efficacy of exogenous surfactant. To my knowledge no one has yet applied this concept in the clinical setting.

Dr. Marini: We have been using ambroxol for many years to enhance surfactant production after birth, at the suggestion of Wauer from Germany. This compound stimulates the production of surfactant by the type 2 pneumocytes. In a multicenter study (2) we found that it reduced the severity of RDS and caused a reduction in mortality. However, the effects are not so dramatic as with surfactant therapy and it takes about 36 h before surfactant-like material appears in tracheal aspirates. It seems possible that it might be beneficial to give both ambroxol and surfactant at birth, so that when the exogenous surfactant is wearing off, the ambroxol stimulation will be taking effect. I do not think glucocorticoids should be used immediately after birth. Experience in the past has shown an increased incidence of IVH. I am also concerned about thyroid hormones because, although you enhance pulmonary maturation, you lower the levels of superoxide dismutase and this may increase the hazard of oxygen toxicity.

I have one further question: What is the clearance rate of your surfactant and is it cleared more slowly than naturally occurring surfactant? This is important in relation to the function of macrophages.

Dr. Fujiwara: The clearance rates of several different surfactant preparations have been extensively studied by Jobe in animal models. His studies show that Surfactant TA (our preparation) stays in the lungs longer than other surfactants. A recent report by Sherman suggests that if pulmonary macrophages are loaded with excess surfactant lipids there may be a reduction in pulmonary host defenses. We have no evidence of increased infection and no other groups have found this either, using different surfactants. However, this is potentially an important issue, and I think at the moment it is best to use the minimum effective dose of good quality surfactant, say 100 mg/kg, to minimize any possible macrophage problem.

REFERENCES

1. Daniels CB, Barr HA, Nicholas TE. A comparison of the surfactant associated lipids derived from reptilian and mammalian lungs. *Respir Physiol* 1989;75:335–48.
2. Marini A, Franzetti M, Gios G, *et al.* Ambroxol in the treatment of idiopathic respiratory distress syndrome. *Respiration* 1987;51(Suppl 1):60–7.

Subject Index